From Ayurveda to Chinese Medicine

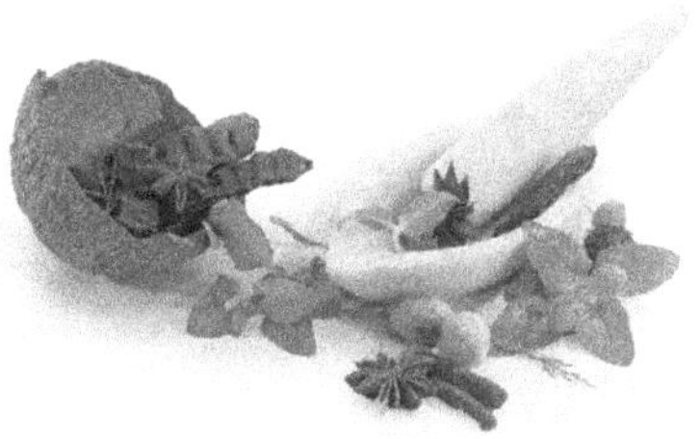
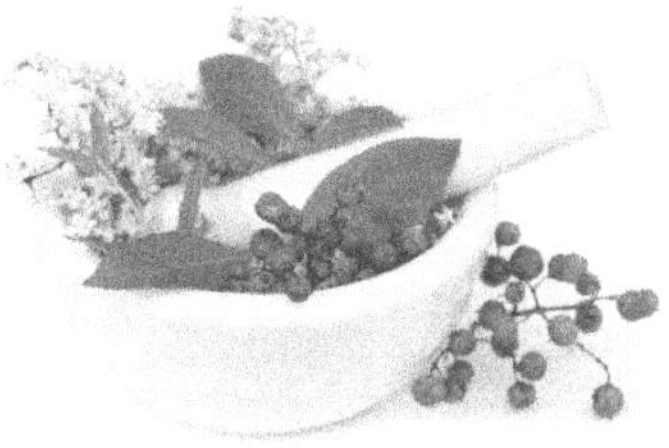

From Ayurveda to Chinese Medicine

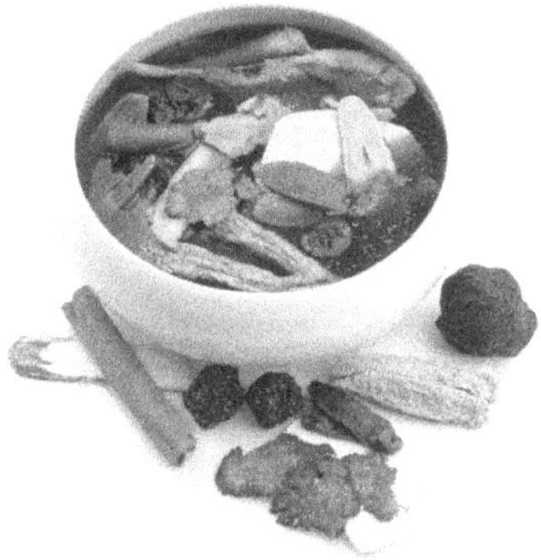

Editors

Ping-Chung Leung
The Chinese University of Hong Kong

Debashis Panda
B.A.M.S.(Gold Medal), M.D.(Gold Medal), D.N.H.E.
Senior Medical Officer
Central Govt. Health Scheme
Govt. of INDIA, New Delhi

World Scientific

NEW JERSEY • LONDON • SINGAPORE • BEIJING • SHANGHAI • HONG KONG • TAIPEI • CHENNAI • TOKYO

Published by

World Scientific Publishing Co. Pte. Ltd.

5 Toh Tuck Link, Singapore 596224

USA office: 27 Warren Street, Suite 401-402, Hackensack, NJ 07601

UK office: 57 Shelton Street, Covent Garden, London WC2H 9HE

Library of Congress Cataloging-in-Publication Data
Names: Leung, Ping-Chung, 1941– editor.
Title: From Ayurveda to Chinese medicine / edited by Ping-Chung Leung.
Description: New Jersey : World Scientific, 2016. | Includes bibliographical references and index.
Identifiers: LCCN 2016039024 | ISBN 9789813200333 (hardcover : alk. paper)
Subjects: | MESH: Medicine, Ayurvedic | Medicine, Chinese Traditional |
Phytotherapy | Complementary Therapies
Classification: LCC R733 | NLM WB 55.A9 | DDC 615.5/38--dc23
LC record available at https://lccn.loc.gov/2016039024

British Library Cataloguing-in-Publication Data
A catalogue record for this book is available from the British Library.

Desk Editors: Suraj Kumar/Joy Quek

Typeset by Stallion Press

Email: enquiries@stallionpress.com

About the Editors

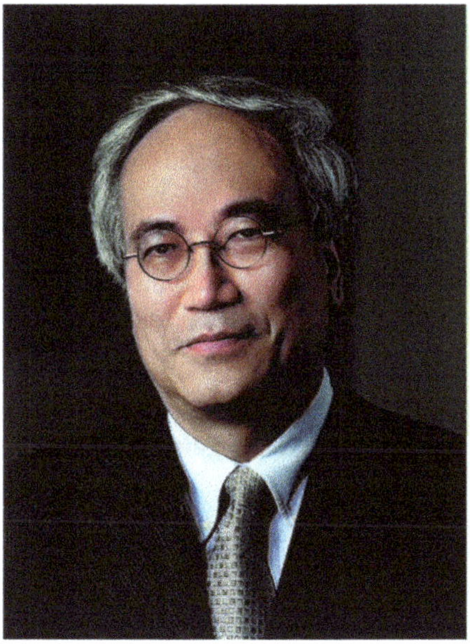

Professor Ping-Chung Leung, OBE, JP, Hon DSSc, DSC, MBBS, MS, FRACS, FRCS(Edin), FHKCOS, FHKAM(Orth); is Emeritus Professor of Orthopaedics & Traumatology, Faculty of Medicine; Director of Centre for Clinical Trials on Chinese Medicine, Institute of Chinese Medicine; Director, The Hong Kong Jockey Club Centre for Osteoporosis Care and Control, The Chinese University of Hong Kong, 1996–2013; Director, Partner State Key Laboratory of Phytochemistry and Plant Resources in West China (The Chinese University of Hong Kong). He is also the Past President of the International Research Society of Orthopaedic Surgery and Traumatology (SIROT), 2009–2012.

Professor Leung's research areas including Orthopaedics, Osteoporosis, Microsurgery, Public Health, Traditional Chinese Medicine (TCM) and General Education. He is also the author of over 800 scientific manuscripts in journals and 27 books. Professor Leung has been appointed as editor of 11 International Journals since 1982. He is trying hard to develop a research methodology basing on modern clinical science requirements, to modernise TCM.

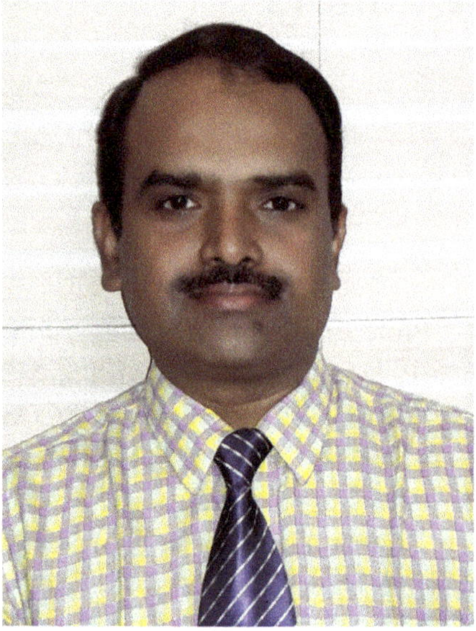

Dr. Debashis Panda is a noted name in the new generation of Ayurveda experts. He has established himself as a distinct persuader of ancient traditional wisdom of Ayurveda in the arena of therapeutics, research and education. He received his M.D. in Dravyaguna Vijnana (Ayurveda Pharmacology) from the National Institute of Ayurveda, Jaipur.

Dr. Debashis Panda was awarded 'Gold Medal' for securing highest marks in the Utkal University and was also honored with 'The Best Thesis Award' during Post Graduation. He has authored books & research papers in several peer reviewed journals. At present, he serves Government of India as a Senior Medical Officer under the Central Government Health Scheme.

List of Contributors

Au Wai-Chun, Edmond
Institute of Chinese Medicine
The Chinese University of Hong Kong, Shatin
New Territories, Hong Kong SAR, PR China

Bahadur, Shiv
School of Natural Product Studies
Department of Pharmaceutical Technology
Jadavpur University, Kolkata 700032, India

Banerjee, Subhadip
School of Natural Product Studies
Department of Pharmaceutical Technology
Jadavpur University, Kolkata 700032, India

Harwansh, Ranjit K
School of Natural Product Studies
Department of Pharmaceutical Technology
Jadavpur University, Kolkata 700032, India

Kar, Amit
School of Natural Product Studies
Department of Pharmaceutical Technology
Jadavpur University, Kolkata 700032, India

Ko, Erik Chun-Hay
Institute of Chinese Medicine
The Chinese University of Hong Kong, Shatin
New Territories, Hong Kong SAR, PR China

Koon, Johnny Chi-Man
Institute of Chinese Medicine
The Chinese University of Hong Kong, Shatin
New Territories, Hong Kong SAR, PR China

Lau, Clara Bik-San
Institute of Chinese Medicine
The Chinese University of Hong Kong, Shatin
New Territories, Hong Kong SAR, PR China

Mukherjee, Pulok K
School of Natural Product Studies
Department of Pharmaceutical Technology
Jadavpur University, Kolkata 700032, India

Yue, Grace Gar-Lee
Institute of Chinese Medicine
The Chinese University of Hong Kong, Shatin
New Territories, Hong Kong SAR, PR China

Contents

Introduction

Ping-Chung Leung

Traditional Indian Medicine Ayurveda and Traditional Chinese Medicine (TCM) are the oldest systems of health care: the former mastering 5,000 years of documentations, the latter at least 3,000 years. All ancient medicine has strong philosophical background and management varieties related to manual activities. Indeed, Ayurveda is strongly linked with Yoga and TCM with activities related to martial art and acupuncture. It is a common belief that in the United States, before Yoga was popularly practised, Ayurveda was hardly known. As for Chinese medicine, acupuncture has been taken as the hallmark. Medicinal herbs, which actually form the main core of treatment in Chinese medicine, were virtually unknown outside China.

Of course, there is a broad background behind which the emerging popularity gradually develops.

Firstly, there is the disillusion about the ever expanding trust over modern medicine. It is true that modern medicine has made marvellous strides within hardly over one century to attain the modern day wonders like organ transplantations, test-tube babies, genomic controls and the rapid emergence of "target therapies". Every epoch making advancement is achieved through a clear understanding about a target to be dealt with followed by the creation of either a promotive or antagonistic agent to flourish or destroy it. The wondrous results have been achieved through thorough understandings of clear-cut, straightforward targets. When results are short of perfection, sometimes even disappointing, in spite of hard efforts, it is often revealed that the target is not simple but complex and poorly understood, so that treatment cannot be satisfactory. Examples are plenty: cancers and aging related degenerations. The cancer patient who faces persistent spread of the cancer would look for traditional medicine (TM). The elderly who is threatened everyday with deteriorating health would wish to try any other option that might help.

It is becoming clear that degenerative diseases and in some other odd situations could be so complicated that causative factors are multiple, unclear and would remain obscure. Trying to remove or control the unknown factors cannot rely on known targets. Modern medicine, in the current context, therefore, can never be perfect.

Secondly, advances in clinical science in the past decades have led to a rapid development of specialisation in the service sector which is expected to provide perfect skills and opportunities. The reliance on technology follows closely in the wide varieties of diagnostic investigations and treatment offers. The overwhelming choices of technical tools to support suggestions on serious diagnoses and to rule out other possibilities have turned suspicions into confirmations. As the need for technological support grows, the human aspect of service provision deteriorates. Investigations are done on demand and to remove doubts which might all lead to over-investigations, unnecessary expenses and loss of human concern and judgment. Disease managements have very much followed the same pathway. Expectations are high, while treatment offers follow either the most optimistic line which could be technology orientated, such as "minimally invasive" or "robotic" approaches. Much satisfaction usually results, intermingling with dissatisfaction. Those dissatisfied would naturally look for alternative possibilities in TM.

Thirdly, it is becoming more and more common for individuals to realise that they are bothered by not one but a number of diseases or ailments. With the exception of only a few who could afford, most people could not help hesitating whether multiple experts should be consulted in order to acquire the best care. Instead, the controversy would remind those involved about the importance of self-care. Ayurveda is giving much recommendations on life style and yoga exercises. Likewise, Chinese medicine has a lot to offer on different forms of exercises and dietary supplements using herbs. What the two ancient health care systems could offer are in fact quite similar in the conceptual context, within which self-care occupies a paramount position.[a]

This book is putting the two systems together to increase the understanding rather than to compare and contrast. For Asians, there must be a natural tendency of personal choice under related cultural influences, so that Indians prefer Ayurveda and Chinese prefer Chinese medicine. The non-Asians, however, would like to understand more about the similarities and differences which would help them to make a personal choice in their pursuit of self-care.

---

[a] Svoboda, R. and Lade, A. (1995). *Tao and Dharma — Chinese Medicine and Ayurveda.* Lotus Press, WI 53181.

Chapter 1

Ayurveda–Chinese Medicine: From Philosophy to Basic Principles

Debashis Panda

Abstract

Towards the end of the 20th Century, modern medicine has become the mainstream of health care in almost all parts of the world. However, in spite of much advances in modern medicine, alternative medicine worldwide still plays an important role in treating the unsolved problems. In some underdeveloped places, it retains its status of being the mainstream treatment. If one looks back into the pre-historical period, he would find four main systems of ancient healing arts. They are: Ayurveda or Indian System of Medicine, Traditional Chinese Medicine (TCM), Ancient Greek Medicine and Egyptian Medicine. One cannot deny the influences: all these primitive practices have existed independently since ancient times. Though all the systems of medicine have unique principles and concepts, there are some similarities also. Geographically, China and India are two adjacent countries, have great influence upon each other in their cultures, religions and medicines. Similar is the case with Greek and Egypt, they also bear some common features. The Greek and Egyptian systems of medicine concentrate on the use of single herbs, while the Chinese and Indian systems rely upon complex preparations. Combined formulae are most frequently prescribed in Chinese and Indian systems of medicine. Of course, Ayurveda and TCM, both seem to be more ancient, their history dating back to 3,000 B.C. (Takakusu, 1956).

In this book, an effort is given to elaborate and compare both ancient systems of medicine in Asia with their philosophies and principles of treatment, so that further scientific research can be carried out in collaboration for the betterment of medical development.

Keywords: Ayurveda; Traditional Chinese Medicine (TCM); *Prakriti–Purush*; *Yin–Yang* Theory; Five-Element Theory.

1.1 Introduction

Both systems of Ayurveda and Chinese medicine consider the patient as a whole instead of treating a particular organ or system as in the case of modern medicine. They regard the human body and its physiological Functions as a selective manifestation of the grand cosmic order. Whatever happens in the human body is a mirror image in minute form of what is happening in the whole universe. The cosmic energies which permeate the whole universe, both animate and inanimate, are also regulating the functioning of human beings. Ancient profounders of Chinese medicine borrowed the concepts and principles directly from traditional Taoist philosophy. Whereas Ayurvedic principles have their root in *Nyāya–Vaiśeşika* and *Sānkhya–Yoga darśanas*, the ancient spiritual philosophies of India. Although, Ayurveda is considered as non man-made, the verses of the Almighty "Brahma" were spontaneously created at the time of origin of the universe.

1.2 *Yin–Yang* versus *Prakriti–Purush*

Yin–Yang is a common Chinese term used simultaneously in both Chinese medicine and Taoist philosophy. *Yin* and *Yang* are regarded as two primordial cosmic forces responsible for all natural phenomena and life processes. These two forces are quite opposite and yet complementary to each other. And it is because of the perfect balance between them that the whole universe remains stable. So, they are interdependent to each other and one cannot exist without the other. Everything in the natural world is constantly under the opposing forces of *Yin* and *Yang* (Yin and Shuai, 1992).

Depending upon their nature and other characteristics, four important aspects in their relationship can be summarised.

1. *Yin* and *Yang* are two opposite but complementary primordial cosmic forces.
2. *Yin* and *Yang* are interdependent, i.e. one cannot exist without the other.
3. Their energies can be transformed from each other (mutual transformation of energy).
4. *Yin* and *Yang* maintain a dynamic equilibrium in the universe, nature and human activities.

Furthermore, the interplay between these two cosmic forces represents the changes and happenings in the universe and also in human activities. *Yin* is the negative or passive force whereas *Yang* symbolises the positive or active force. The differences in their characteristics can be categorised as follows:

Yin	*Yang*
Female	Male
Negative	Positive
Passive force	Active force
Darkness	Brightness
Low-lying	High-flying
Conversing	Expanding
Descending	Ascending
Heavy	Light
Earth	Heaven

The *Yin–Yang* theory permeates entirely into all spheres of Chinese medicine. Good health is considered as an equilibrium of these two opposite forces and diseases develop, when this equilibrium is disturbed. All the structural components and functional activities of the body are divided into two groups — *Yin* and *Yang*. The diagnosis, the treatment principles, selection of herbs, composition of herbs, forms of administration are all based on the *Yin–Yang* theory (Cai *et al.*, 1995).

Similarly, the *Prakriti–Purush* concept of Ayurveda and primeval philosophies of ancient India depict the theory of evolution of modern scientists. *Prakriti* is known as *Moola Prakriti* or primordial entity, known also as the cosmic egg, and its other synonym is *Avyakta* i.e. Unmanifested Matter. *Moola Prakriti* or primordial entity is a composite unit of three properties, which can be seen as three cosmic energies or forces.

They are:

Sattva = Force of balance,
Raja = Force of activate,
Tama = Force of conserve.

These three forces are mutually interdependent and are never found in isolation from one another. Unless and until their balanced state is disturbed, they remain as inert and static. However, when one force starts to dominate the other two, ultimately the state of equilibrium is disturbed. Thereafter, the concentrated mass of primordial entity i.e. *Moola Prakriti* would burst out violently, followed by the delivery of five cosmic elements (i.e. *Panchbhutas*). This may be equivalent to what modern astronomists called the Big Bang. These five cosmic elements in turn constitute various objects of this universe, both animate and inanimate. Since everything in this universe is part of *Moola Prakriti* or primordial entity, everything should possess the three primitive properties — *sattva, raja, tama* i.e. the three cosmic energies (Filliozat, 1964).

The classical descriptions commonly used to denote the difference between *Prakriti* and *Purush* are as follows:

Prakriti	*Purush*
One	More
Achetana (unconscious)	*Chetana* (conscious)
Triguna (three properties)	*Aguna* (no properties)
Beejadharmini	*Abeejadharma*
Prasavadharmini	*Aprasavadharma*
Amadhyasthadharmini	*Madhyasthadharma*
Female	Male

The three words, namely, *Beejadharmini*, *Prasavadharmini* and *Madhyasthadharmini* are most important. *Beejadharmini* means *Moola Prakriti* has all the substances of this universe in subtle form inside; very much like the seed containing the whole tree inside it. *Prasavadharmini* means *Moola Prakriti* has the ability of delivery of cosmic particles for the evolution of universe. The explosion of cosmic egg with a large bang can be correlated with the painful cry of a mother during delivery. *Amadhyasthadharmini*, means there is no resting phase for the primordial body: Evolution and Dissolution is a continuous process without any resting phase. At the time of dissolution, this materialistic universe first disintegrates into cosmic elements, which again form the primordial body or *Moola Prakriti*. This is not a surprising fact because in the course of astronomical time, the black holes in the universe will swallow all nearby celestial bodies and thereafter will attract one another to form aggregated masses, which will develop into cosmic eggs. Another synonym of *Moola Prakriti* is *Brahmanda*, which consists of two words, *Brahma* + *Anda*. Here, *Brahma* means huge and *Andam* means egg. So, *Brahmanda* literally means the cosmic egg. The aggregated primordial body will have plenty of cosmic energies, which can be divided into three forms, i.e. balancing, activating and conversing energies, which are *sattva*, *raja*, and *tama* respectively. These cosmic energies will maintain an equilibrium till the next evolution takes place and the same procedures will repeat when evolution starts (Heyn, 1987).

Based on such considerations, it is now essential to know what *Purush* is and what is its role in the origin of universe and life. From the definition, it is clear that *Purush* is the conscious subject, who always remains in the resting phase and is unlimited in number. *Purush* is not directly responsible for the evolution process because the process of evolution is automatic. Yet, *Purush* is considered as the creator in Hindu philosophy. As *Purush* is conscious, it is responsible for Life. Every living object in this universe has an individual soul, hence, *Purush* can be considered as the Supreme Soul or Universal Soul (Zummer, 1948).

The entire phenomena can be represented as follows:

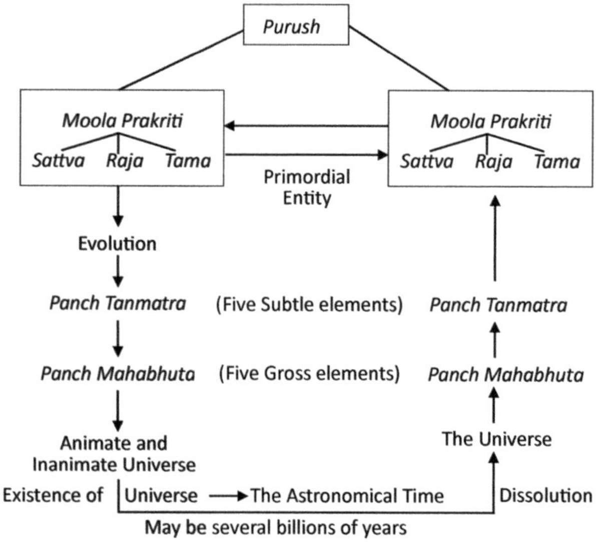

1.3 Relation of *Yin–Yang* Theory to Health and Longevity

Yin–Yang forces exist everywhere, starting from the universe to minute cells of the human body. There are always interactions between these two cosmic forces within the body and also between the body and the environment. The dynamic equilibrium of these two forces in the body is the indicator of good health and prolonged longevity. Disease occurs when this balance is disturbed which may be due to an excess or deficiency of any of these two forces under internal or environmental influences. Preventive medicine has been given more importance in Traditional Chinese Medicine (TCM) since ancient times and this can only be achieved by maintaining the balance between *Yin* and *Yang* through proper diet and exercise with careful attention to changes is season and weather. Dietary regimen and physical activities can be modified according to different seasons and sometimes herbal medicines are also given to replenish the deficiency.

Structural components and functional activities of the body are classified into *Yin* and *Yang* categories though nothing is absolute about *Yin* or *Yang* inside the body. Indeed, the dominance of *Yin* or *Yang* is always relative. A general classification of *Yin* and *Yang* is given in the following table.

Yin	*Yang*
Internal body	External body surface
Lower part of body	Upper part of body
Front portion of body	Back portion of body
Medial aspect of body	Lateral aspect of body
Solid (*zang*) organs	Hollow (*fu*) organs
Governs blood & body fluids	Governs *Qi* (energy)
Body vessels	*Qi* Meridians
Innate instincts	Learned skills
Woman	Man

Woman is considered *Yin* and Man as *Yang* but both man and woman are under the influence of both principles. Similarly, each organ is under the influence of both forces and it is the dominance of *Yin* or *Yang* within that organ or body part that gives the decisive influence. Taoists believe that *Yin* is preferred to *Yang*. However, both forces are equally important for good health and longevity (Beinfield and Korngold, 1991).

The basic principle of treatment is to restore the balance between *Yin* and *Yang*. Since both are opposite and complementary to each other, when *Yin* increases *Yang* decreases and *vice versa*. The possible states of imbalance resulting from their disturbed equilibrium are:

(i) An absolute excess in *Yin* leading to a recession in *Yang*.
(ii) An absolute excess in *Yang* leading to a recession in *Yin*.
(iii) A relative increase in *Yin* due to deficiency in *Yang*.
(iv) A relative increase in *Yang* due to deficiency in *Yin*.

Under the above conditions, it is essential to redress the imbalance by expelling out the excess and supplementing the deficiency. When the imbalance is mild, body automatically corrects it. But when it crosses the limit, medication and other means are needed to restore the balance.

Similar principles are found in Ayurveda for maintaining the balance in the body. *Soma–Agni* principle of Ayurveda is almost the same to the above consideration, where *Soma* means water and *Agni* means fire. To redress the imbalance, food and medicines of *Sheeta veerya* (cold potency) and *Ushna veerya* (hot potency) are administered. When there is excess cold (*Soma tattva*), drugs of hot potency are given. Similarly, in excessive hot conditions, food and medicines of cold potency are prescribed.

1.4 The Theory of the Five Elements

Both ancient systems of medicine believe that every structure of this universe including the human body (body parts, organs, tissues, cells, etc.), plants, animals, and other substances are composed of five elements. Interaction of these five elements, their balanced relationships and unions are responsible for the existence of this materialistic universe. The physiological state, pathological state and the treatment are all dependent on the five-element theory. Although both TCM and Ayurveda consider the five-element theory in their concept and principles, they differ in the basic explanation of these five cosmic elements. The differences are as follows:

TCM	Ayurveda
Wood	Space (*Akash*)
Fire	Air (*Vayu*)
Earth	Fire (*Agni*)
Metal	Water (*Jala*)
Water	Earth (*Prithvi*)

Fire, water and earth are the same in both systems of medicine. TCM takes wood and metal as two components of the five elements whereas Ayurveda includes space and air. Furthermore, the concept and application of the five-element theory differ in both ancient systems with some similarities. The concepts are unique and complete within themselves. It is necessary to study the concepts separately in their respective ways and later evaluate the similarities and dissimilarities in further research (Bensky and Gamble, 1993; O'Brien, 2002).

1.5 Five-Element Theory in Ayurveda

For the complete understanding of the five-element theory, i.e. *Panch Mahabhuta* theory in Ayurveda, it is essential to know the evolution sequence along with the formation of animate and inanimate universe.

First of all, it is important to know how these five cosmic elements are evolved. As discussed previously, everything is originated from the primordial entity (*Moola Prakriti*). From the primordial entity the five cosmic elements are evolved, which later constitute the whole universe by combining with one another in varied proportions. Everything is composed of five elements, but it is only the different proportions that the different structures are unique in their shape, size, quality and activities. There are two schools of thought regarding the evolution of five elements (*Panch Mahabhutas*). The first theory is that all the five elements are evolved simultaneously and independently from their respective subtle forms (*Panch Tanmatra*). In the second school of thought, it is assumed that the five elements have evolved one from the other i.e. air from space, fire from air, water from fire and earth from water. The second school of thought seems more logical and it was admitted by most of the ancient sages. Most theories about the origin of the earth assume that it began in a gaseous state, evolved to a liquid state and finally became partly solid (Encyclopaedia Britannica, 1980). Similar types of assumptions are made long before by Ayurveda sages and also found in Indian philosophy. Here, Air and Fire are correlated with gaseous state, water represents liquid state and earth represents solid state. Space is the most primitive one from which evolution of the five elements started. In the evolution of the five elements, there is an intermediate state of subtle five elements, which directly evolved from the primordial entity and later develop into the gross five elements. These gross five elements, their interactions and their composition in varied proportions are responsible for the creation of the materialistic world.

So, there are three physical states of the five elements known as *Panch Mahabhutas* found. They are:

(i) Subtler state or atomic state: *Sukhma Bhutas* or *Paramanu.*
(ii) Molecular state or subtle state: *Pithara* or *Anu Stage.*
(iii) Material state or gross state: *Drishya bhutas.*

Drishya Bhutas, the last material state, is the aggregate of molecules, *pitharas* of the same element or different elements at varied proportions. This state is visible to naked eyes but the previous two states are invisible. It is a surprising fact that the ancient sages of Ayurveda appear to know about the atomic theory (atom — *Paramanu*, molecule — *Pithara*) much earlier before.

1.6 Evolution of the Five Elements

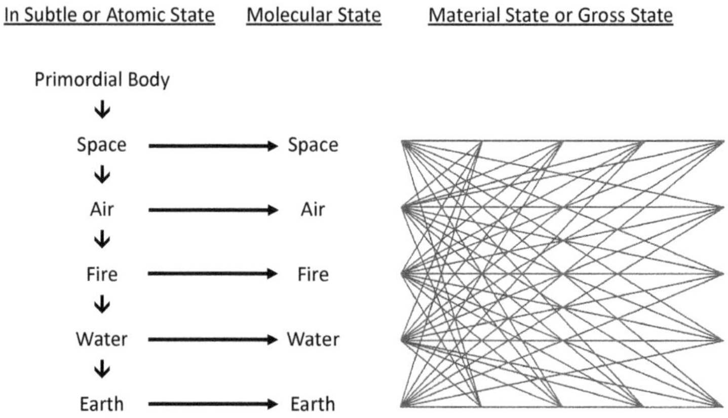

Early scholars of Ayurveda advocated nine basic elements or causative elements: *Karana dravyas*, which includes the five elements described above for the creation of animate and inanimate materials. The other four elements are: soul (*Ātma*), mind (*Mana*), time (*Kala*), and direction (*Dik*). The five elements are directly involved in the formation of matters whereas the latter four elements, which do not have any physical form, are indirectly involved. The other four elements are not accepted by modern scientists to date as to be involved in the formation of different matters (Raina, 1990).

1.7 Five-Element Theory versus Atomic Theory

The ancient five-element theory can be correlated with the atomic theory of modern science as follows:

Five elements		Atomic structure
Space	Empty space	Where electrons move
Air	Kinetic energy	Movement of the electrons resembling the solar system or other celestial bodies in universe
Fire	Heat energy or electric charge	Negative charged electron and positive charged proton. Positron having one positive charge

(*Continued*)

(*Continued*)

Five elements		Atomic structure
Water	Force of cohesion	Centripetal and centrifugal force created due to movement of electrons around the nucleus
Earth	Mass of the atom	The nucleus — proton and neutron

Atom is the smallest and the least dynamic division of an element or material and so is the cell to a living organism. An atom of an element is responsible for the chemical and physical properties of that element and similarly the biological cell of a living organism is responsible for the physiological activities. Scholars of Ayurveda use the concept of the five elements, the *Panch Mahabhuta* theory, to know the properties and actions of different objects and also the physiological functions of organs and body tissues.

Cell of Living Organism

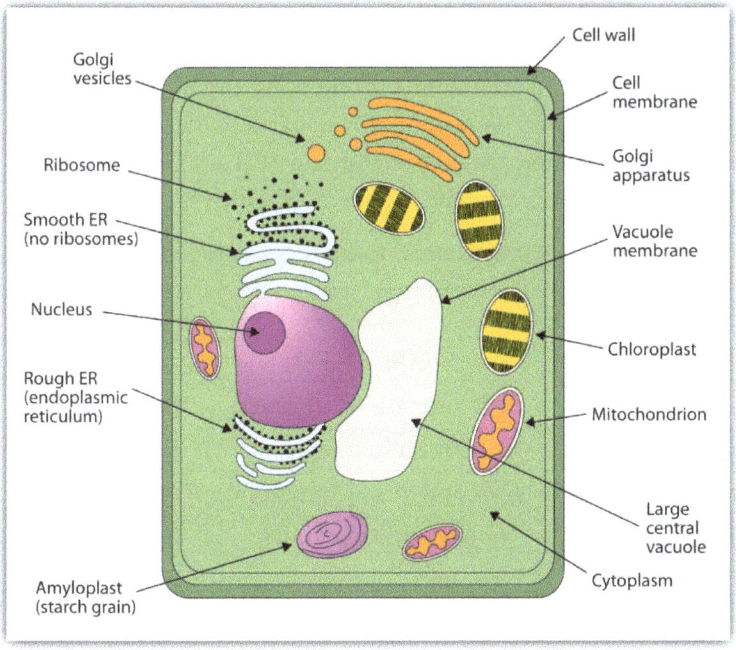

1.8 Body Parts Attributed to the Five Elements

No part of the body is attributed absolutely to any of the five elements. However, different parts of the body are categorised under the five elements depending upon the predominance. As discussed above, every part, organ and tissue is made up of all the five elements combined at different proportions.

Space — Empty spaces, differentiation of body cells, tissues, organs, etc. from one another. Empty spaces of external opening like ear, nose, mouth, etc. External, middle and internal ear with conduction of sound waves and instrument of hearing.

Air — Act of respiration and excretion, contraction, expansion and voluntary and involuntary movements of body part. Feeling of touch and the whole skin with touch receptors are controlled by Air.

Fire — Helps in digestion, assimilation and complete metabolism process. Responsible for complexion and lustre. Functions of eyes and act of vision are governed by fire.

Water — Governs all the fluid media of the body: blood, plasma, lymph, mucus secretions, etc. Urine, sweat, fat, are also controlled. Tongue with taste buds and the system of taste perception are controlled by water.

Earth — Earth provides shape and form of the body and is responsible for the stability, heaviness and hardness.

Body structures like bone, teeth, muscles, organs, tendons and ligaments are all composed predominantly of earth. Nose, smell receptors and mechanism of smelling are governed by earth (Lad, 1990).

We have five sensory organs and each of which is controlled by one of the five elements.

Five elements	Sensory sense	Sense organ	Function
Space	Sound	Ears and auditory system	Hearing
Air	Touch	Skin and touch receptor	Feeling of touch
Fire	Sight	Eyes and visual system	Act of seeing
Water	Taste	Tongue and taste buds	Perception of taste
Earth	Smell	Nose and olfactory system	Act of smelling

From the previous discussions, it is clear that the five elements: *Panch Mahabhutas* are evolved from the primordial entity (*Moola Prakriti*) and from the five elements, everything in this universe, both animate and inanimate are created. Therefore, the five elements including human beings, animals, vegetables, foods, drinks, etc. are characterised by the three properties: *sattva, raja, tama* — the three cosmic forces of primordial entity, *Moola Prakriti*. Everything exhibits the three properties of force or energy, but depending upon the predominance, the object is named and functions accordingly. In summary, the three forces are:

Sattva = Force of balance (that balances the other two forces).
Raja = Force of activation.
Tama = Force of conserve.

The five elements are composed predominantly of:

Space = *Sattva* = Force of balance.
Air = *Raja* = Force of activation.
Fire = *Sattva* + *Raja* = Force of balance and activation.
Water = *Sattva* + *Tama* = Force of balance and conserve.
Earth = *Tama* = Force of conserve.

Everything in this world is composed of five elements, *Panch Mahabhutas*, and so are the foods and medicines. After digestion, absorption and assimilation, foods and medicines augment their respective homologous structures in the body. In the process of digestion, foods and medicines get broken down into five distinct physico-chemical groups of five elements and process to augment the corresponding elements that compose the human body. This has a parallel correlation in modern concept that oxygen loss can only be replenished by oxygen derived from the environment or outside sources. Similarly, the other chemical elements like sodium, potassium, calcium, iron, magnesium, iodine, copper, zinc, selenium, and vitamins, proteins, etc. need to be supplied through food and supplements in case of deficiency. Substances, similar in terms of form, quality and action contribute to an increase of these corresponding constituents in the body and dissimilar substances are responsible for the decrease of those corresponding constituents. This is the fundamental principle which serves as the basic of Ayurveda treatment (*Sāmānya-viśesha Siddhānta*).

Variable composition of the five elements in a substance is responsible for the existence of different tastes in it. There are six primary tastes considered in Ayurveda, in contrast to the five tastes in Chinese medicine and four in modern human physiology. Variable composition of tastes in food and medicine are responsible for the different pharmacological activities. Drugs having more than one taste or having more tastes are capable of performing a number of biological effects in the body. The six tastes and their compositions in relation to the five elements are as follows:

Tastes	Composition	Potency
Madhura = Sweet	Earth + Water	Cold
Amla = Sour (or acid)	Earth + Fire	Hot
Lavana = Salt (or saline)	Water + Fire	Hot
Katu = Pungent (or acrid)	Air + Fire	Hot
Tikta = Bitter	Air + Space	Cold
Kashaya = Astringent	Air + Earth	Cold

1.9 Concept of the Three Humours

In further continuation, the five elements contribute towards the three humours in the body which are responsible for the body physiology and meta-physical activities. The three humours are — *vata*, *pitta* and *kapha*. Each of the three humours is not influenced by all the five elements. Rather, one or two of the five elements constitute a humour. So, the humours can be considered functional units of the five elements in the body. The five-element theory and the three humour theory are complementary to each other, but in general, the practice of the three humour theory is more popular and more frequently used in treatment planning. The first two elements unite to form *vata*, the middle element constitutes *pitta* and the last two elements combine together to form *kapha*. However, *vata* is more active in nature (*Raja bahulya*), *pitta* is more balancing (*Sattva bahulya*) and *kapha* is more conserving in nature (*Tama bahulya*).

Vata = Space + Air = Activative or dynamic in nature.
Pitta = Fire = Balancing or transformative in nature.
Kapha = Water + Earth = Conserving or stabilising in nature.

The three humours are influenced collectively by the five elements but are not composed of the five elements individually. Rather, it can be considered that the five elements are divided into three categories to become the three humours. The three humours reside in every cell in subtle form as the cells are composed of five elements. The three humours are responsible for all the physiological and pathological activities of the human body. As long as the three humours maintain in equilibrium, good health continues and when they fail to achieve the state of equilibrium, disease occurs. They may be increased or decreased compared with their normal levels, thus becoming diseased. The duty of the physician is to lower the increased humours, or increase the decreased humour, pacify the overactive humours, redress the balance and control the pathological activities. Being in constant circulation through out the body, they regulate the life activities of the body (Udupa and Singh, 1978).

In modern terms, these three humours can be correlated with the neurohormones of modern science. Neurohormones are biochemical substances secreted by the nerve endings and endocrine glands; they activate body tissues and organs in day-to-day function. Biochemists believe that the biochemicals like adrenaline, noradrenaline, acetylcholine, prostaglandins, histamine, etc. are the play masters of the body organs. These biochemicals are secreted under different situations and are responsible for body physiology, pathology and related changes. Ayurveda experts believe that the functions of the three humours go beyond the levels of activities of biochemicals. They concentrate on the conditions which are responsible for the secretion of these biochemicals. In other words, they control the secretion of biochemicals. Biochemicals or neurohumours are the materialistic form of the three humours formed in extra-cellular space, which control different physiological and pathological activities of the human body. So, the three humours, which presumably are intracellular could be studied more scientifically in line with the discovery of molecular biology in modern biological science.

However, in Ayurveda the three humours can be understood for practical applications in treatment planning as follows:

Vata: Activities of nervous system (both sympathetic and parasympathetic).
Mental: Enthusiasm, concentration, happiness or sadness.
Physical: Respiration, circulation, excretion and every type of voluntary action.

Pitta: Activities of enzymes and hormones.
Mental: Intellect, clear conception.
Physical: Digestion and metabolism, nutrition, thermo-genesis and tissue building and skin lustre.

Kapha: Activities of tissue fluid and skeletal system, process of anabolism.
Mental: Courage, tolerance, power of retention of memory.
Physical: Body, strength, immunity, tissue building, joint function, gland secretions.

These three humours are again sub-divided into five divisions each. These sub-divisions will be discussed at appropriate places later in this book.

1.10 Five-Element Theory in Chinese Medicine

In Chinese medicine, the human body is considered a microcosm of the grand cosmic order and is believed to be composed of the five cosmic elements. The five-element theory seems to be interwoven into every aspect of Chinese medicine. Everything in this world is evolved from the five cosmic elements due to their interactions with each other. The five elements exist everywhere, even in the smallest particle of a substance. The five elements are always in dynamic motion and are responsible for the different activities of the world. Nevertheless, they remain in a state of equilibrium with one another. The five elements, their nature and qualities are briefly described as follows:

The five elements (Yin and Shuai, 1992)		
Fire	Warm or hot	Flaring, ascending
Earth	Nourishing	Growing, promoting
Wood	Germination	Growth, flourishing
Metal	Descending	Clearing, astringing
Water	Cooling	Down flowing

The five elements are considered at different stages of human life and could be comfortably compared with the seasonal cycles, day and night, and their continuum. In Chinese medicine, there are four seasons. In contrast, in Ayurveda, six seasons are considered. The normal seasons are Spring, Summer, Autumn and Winter. But in Ayurveda, Rainy and Early Winter (Hemanta) seasons are described (Udupa and Singh, 1978). Sometimes, for the purpose of treatment planning, one more season is considered in Ayurveda: the Early Rainy season (*Pravrit*). Comparing the five elements with the stages of seasonal changes and daily changes, the following tabulation is prepared:

Five elements	Seasonal change	Daily change	Climatic condition
Wood	Spring	Morning	Wind + Warm
Fire	Summer	Midday	Heat (too hot)
Earth	Late summer	Afternoon	Dampness (less hot, moisture)
Metal	Autumn	Sunset	Dryness (cool)
Water	Winter	Midnight	Cold

1.11 Comparison of the Five Elements with Stages of Human Life (Maciocia, 1989)

Five elements	Human life
Wood	Birth and rapid growth in childhood
Fire	Adulthood
Earth	Mature man
Metal	Stage of ageing and degeneration
Water	Stage of hospice and return to a state of dissolution

1.12 Comparison of Seasonal and Daily Changes, between Chinese Medicine and Ayurveda

Daily changes	Season in Chinese medicine	Season in Ayurveda
Morning	Spring	Spring
Midday	Summer	Summer
Afternoon	Late summer	Early rainy
Sunset	Autumn	Rainy
Mid-night	Winter	Autumn
Sunrise	—	Winter

Five elements	Directions
Wood	East
Fire	South
Earth	Centre
Metal	West
Water	North

There are five solid (*Wu zang*) and six hollow (*Liu fu*) organs described in Chinese medicine. The five elements are related to *zang* and *fu* which react to their influence with regard to their physiological and pathological states. The five solid organs are heart, liver, spleen, kidney and lungs and the six hollow organs are gall bladder, stomach, large intestine, small intestine, urinary bladder and "triple warmer", i.e. the openings of stomach, small intestine and bladder combinedly. The interrelationship between the five elements and the *zang–fu* organs provides the basic background to the understanding of the physiological and pathological conditions of the body. The solid and hollow organs are again interrelated and form five coupled pairs. Solid organs are considered to have *Yin* energy whereas hollow organs have *Yang* energy. So, each pair consists of a solid *Yin* organ and a corresponding hollow *Yang* organ and the pair is controlled by one of the five elements. Five sensory senses and five types of body tissues are also composed of the five elements and their functions are controlled by the movement of these five elements inside the body. The interrelationship of body organs with the five elements is depicted below in the following table:

Five elements	Solid organ	Hollow organ	Five sense	Five tissues	Body complexion	Body odour
Wood	Liver	Gall bladder	Eye	Tendons	Green	Rancid
Fire	Heart	Small intestine	Tongue	Blood vessels	Red	Scorched
Earth	Spleen	Stomach	Mouth	Muscles	Yellow	Fragrant
Metal	Lung	Large intestine	Nose	Skin	White	Goatish
Water	Kidney	Urinary bladder	Ears	Bones	Black	Putrid

The body organs and tissues are interrelated and their functions reflect the activities of the five elements. If pathology exists in one of the organ, then the respective group also becomes affected and the relationship with the five elements needs to play a major role in subsequent rectification (Ross, 1985).

At the same time, the five elements and internal organs are associated with mental faculties. Experts in Chinese medicine believe that mental emotions have influence on the physical condition of the body. Both physical and mental needs should be included while treatment is being planned. The solid *Yin* organs are generally associated with the emotions. They also house the five human attributes like spirit, human soul, animal soul, mind and will power. There are five types of primary tastes considered in Chinese medicine (in Ayurveda, there are six tastes) and each one is intimately related to one of the five elements. In addition, five types of fruits and grains are also considered to have connection with the five elements and the *zang–fu* organs. The five elements and *Yin* organs and their relation with mental activities are given in the following table:

Five elements	*Yin* organs	Emotions	Attributes	Sound	Function
Wood	Liver	Anger depression	Human soul*	Shouting	Planning and decision making
Fire	Heart	Joy	Spirit	Laughing	Mood and clarity of thought
Earth	Spleen	Desire, over thinking	Mind	Singing	Concentration
Metal	Lung	Worry	Animal soul*	Crying	Energetic and active
Water	Kidney	Fear	Will power	Groaning	Sexual function and thinking, stick to decision

*Human soul — enters the foetus at the time of birth; Animal soul — enters the embryo at the time of fertilization.

1.13 Relation of Five Elements with Taste, Fruit and Grain

Five elements	Taste	Fruit	Grain
Wood	Sour	Plum	Wheat
Fire	Bitter	Apricot	Glutinous rice
Earth	Sweet	Date	Millet
Metal	Pungent	Pear	Rice
Water	Salt	Chestnut	Pea

The most important aspect of the five-element theory, that is widely practised in treatment of Chinese medicine, is the interrelationship between the five elements. In normal physiological conditions, there exists two cycles. One is the generative cycle from Mother to Offspring sequence and the other is the Subjugative Restraining Cycle (Vector Vanquished sequence). It is believed that each cosmic force of the five elements has both generative and subjugative influences individually and upon one another, thus contributing towards good health or ill health.

1.13.1 *Generative Cycle (Mother to Offspring Sequence)*

As the offspring gets nourishment and support from the mother, each one of the five elements in the cycle, wood–fire–earth–metal–water–wood gets support accordingly. Thus, each element gets nourishment and support from its predecessor. In other words, each element is generated by the previous element and later in turn generates the next one in the cycle. This continues in a cycle, for example: wood generates fire, fire generates earth, earth generates metal, metal generates water, water generates wood, wood again generates fire and the cycle goes on. Literally, it can be understood as follows: Fire corresponds to the state of Hot Liquid at the time of evolution, which cools down to generate earth, by further cooling, some part of earth turns into hard stone and metals, thus generates metal (inanimate world), metals or mountains burst to create rivers (water), water promotes growth of plants, thereby generates wood and the animate world, wood burns to generate fire (at the time of dissolution, everything is destroyed to form the primordial body).

1.13.2 *Subjugative Cycle (Vector Vanquished Sequence)*

In this relationship, each element is controlled by the previous element and it controls the next one. In the sequence of wood–earth–water–fire–metal–wood, earth is vanquished by wood but is victor over fire and so on. Literally, it can be understood as follows: Plants germinate by breaking the earth and then, their roots controls the soil loss by strongly attaching to it, earth controls water by containing it in one place, water subjugates fire by extinguishing it, fire subjugates metal by melting it, and metal controls wood by being heavier than it and cutting it.

Each one of the five elements is associated with a pair of internal organs — one solid *Yin* and another hollow *Yang*. The fundamental relations between the five elements provide the insight to understand the interaction of internal organs and their influence upon one another.

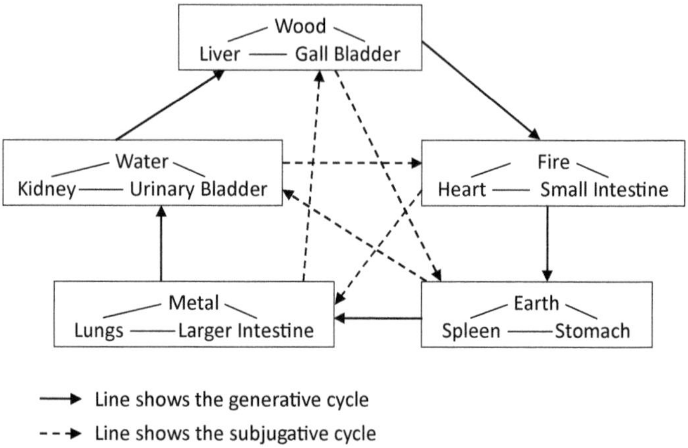

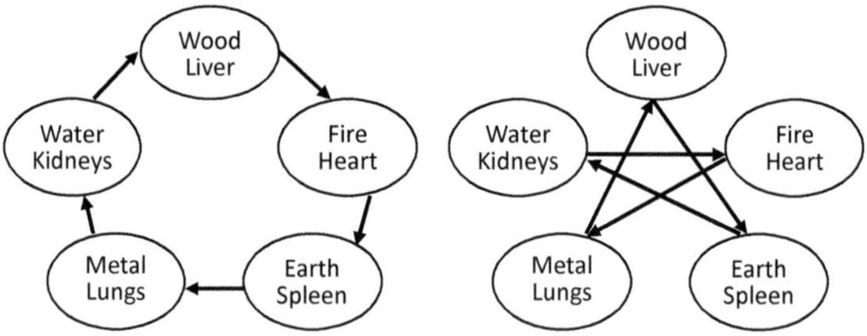

Generative Sequence
(Mother → Offspring Relationship)

Subjugative Sequence
(Victor → Vanquished Relationship)

Clinically, these principles are used as guiding tools both in diagnosis and treatment. In normal physiological state, the organs provide nourishment and support to the next one in the sequence and simultaneously get the nourishment from the previous one. The generative sequence is liver–heart–spleen–lungs–kidneys–liver. So, in the pathological state, if there is problem in the heart, then liver reinforcing herbs are prescribed along with heart strengthening herbs. Similarly, if there is excess in kidneys, then drugs which will inhibit the function of lungs are prescribed. Furthermore, the subjugative sequence is liver–spleen–kidneys–heart–lungs–liver, where the organs are controlled by the previous one and control the next one in the sequence. So, in case of excess urination, spleen and stomach tonifying herbs are given along with lung inhibitory medicines.

Due to deficiency and excess of *zang–fu* (solid–hollow) organs, another two conditions arise in the subjugative sequence. If the previous organ is more efficient and next one is weakened, then the previous organ will over-control the next one and the functions of next organ will be diminished. It is called "overacting" condition in the same subjugative sequence. For example, if the kidneys are overacting the heart, (the condition of heart failure due to kidney pathology), then medicine must be given to calm the kidneys along with heart reinforcing herbs.

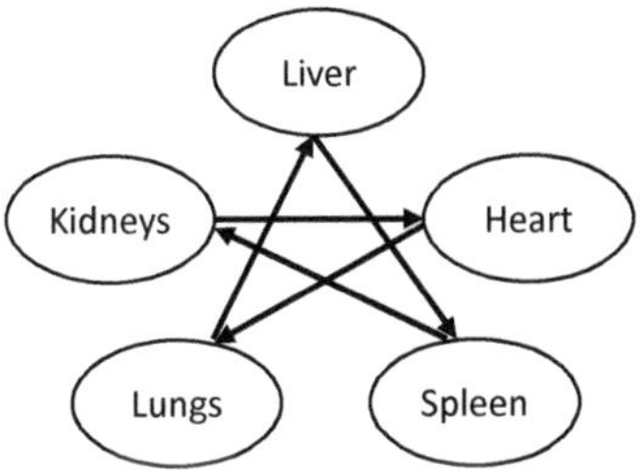

Overacting stage in subjugative sequence

Similarly, another condition arises, when the previous organ becomes weakened and the next organ becomes more active in the subjugative sequence. Thereupon, the next organ starts controlling the previous one, which is just opposite to the normal sequence. This condition is known as stage of "counter-action". These conditions are seen in chronic conditions and are more difficult and take longer to cure. For example, if the spleen is counteracting liver, then the following steps are to be followed to implement the cure.

(i) Calm the spleen by controlling the over-function. Heart tranquilising medicines can be given because the heart is the mother to spleen in the generative sequence.
(ii) Strengthening the liver by liver toning herbs. Kidney toning medicines can be given because liver is the offspring to mother kidney in the generative sequence.
(iii) Regulation of the sequence, so that liver can control spleen again.

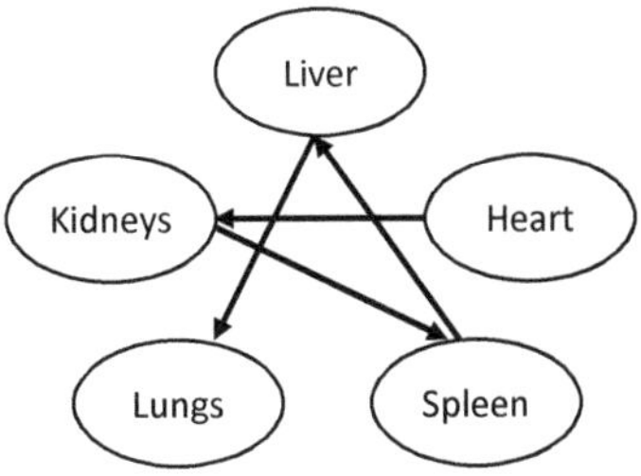

Stage of counter-action in subjugative sequence

Some pathological condition may arise in the generative sequence also. Disorders of the previous organ may transmit to the next organ in the sequence and *vice versa.* (Mother affecting the offspring and offspring affecting the mother.) Both the generative and subjugative sequences are complimentary to each other. The physician has to consider both sequences and possible interactions to reach a final diagnosis or treatment plan.

1.14 Concept of Mind

The definition of health as stated by World Health Organization (WHO, 7 April 1948) is perhaps the most widely accepted definition of health today. It states that, "Health is a state of complete physical, mental and social well-being and not merely the absence of disease or infirmity". Much before the inclusion of mental health in connection with physical health, the most ancient systems of health care; Ayurveda and Chinese medicine, already emphasised the interaction between the body and mind in their old classics almost 5,000 years ago. Mind and body are seen neither separate nor identical but as a continuum, complementary to each other. There would be no complete physical health without good mental health, and *vice versa.* Different mental states and emotions have significant impact on the physical body and *vice versa.* Both Ayurveda and Chinese medicine view body–mind as one system and the dynamic internal equilibrium between them, and their harmony with nature externally are essential for good health. Imbalance is the cause of ill health. The balance between the human beings with nature and surroundings, harmonious ecology and social relationship forms the basis of social and economic productive life. Furthermore, experts of Ayurveda advocate for spiritualism in addition to body–mind harmony for the state of complete health. Chinese medicine does not include the importance of soul in complete health. In spite of that, human soul and animal soul are considered connected with the heart, liver and lungs. Animal soul enters the embryo at the time of conception and human soul enters the foetus at the time of birth.

According to WHO, there is no one official definition of mental health. It is an unarguable fact that the mind plays a vital role in various psychological and physiological activities in the human body. Emotions like anxiety, stress, fear, anger, love, sympathy, envy, greediness are attributes of the mind, which trigger releases of neurotransmitters, which ultimately affect the physiological status of body.

1.14.1 *In Ayurveda*

1. Mind itself has no life, but in association with life (soul) it becomes activated and controls the sensory organs and motor organs.
2. Mind is the super sense organ i.e. it cannot be perceived by the sense organs. Yet, it controls the five sense organs (auditory, skin, vision, gustatory and olfactory) and five motor organs (speech, functions of hands, functions of leg, anus, penis (genitalia) — their centres in brain). This means the perception of sensory senses (sound, touch, vision, taste and smell) and function of motor organs (talking, movement of hands, legs, excretion, sexual act) are only possible when there is presence of the mind in them.
3. Mind is subtle in nature. This means its ability to imagine and reach everywhere. It can travel millions of miles in fraction of a second.
4. Mind is one and only that connects with one sense organ at one time. For examples, if one sees something, then at the same time he/she cannot hear anything. If one tastes something, then at the same time he cannot smell anything. But, we cannot differentiate these actions and usually think they are occurring simultaneously. In fact, these actions are occurring one after another in very quick succession, taking fractions of a second. This is possible due to subtleness of mind for which it switches over to one another in quick intervals. But, there is no two or more minds in a same physical body to be connected with two or more sense organs at the same time.
5. Function of the mind is to control the sense organs and motor organs. It initiates the sense organs in their respective actions and also prevents them from doing so. Along with that, it has the action of self-control, so that it prevents itself from engaging in a particular action.
6. Mind is the organ responsible for thinking. It includes simple thinking, imaginary thinking, inquiring, comparing, speculation, concentration and determination.
7. Location of the mind in the physical body is a controversial topic in Ayurveda. Maximum references are found, where location of the mind

is attributed to heart, while other references include brain, and the structure between soft palate and head. From textual references of Ayurveda, the following three structures may be considered as the site of mind.

A. Heart — Maximum references are found.
B. Brain — With some references.
C. The structure in between head and soft palate, possibly the pineal body (Udupa and Singh, 1978).

In TCM, Mind is thought to be located in Spleen, nevertheless different emotions are also attributed to other internal (Zang) organs. The overall functioning of Mind can be viewed as follows:

Internal organs	Houses	Function	Emotions
Liver	Human soul*	Planning and decision making	Anger, depression
Heart	Spirit	Mood and clarity of thought	Joy
Spleen	Mind	Concentration	Desire, over thinking
Lungs	Animal soul*	Energetic and active	Worry
Kidneys	Will power	Sexual function, thinking and stick to decision	Fear

*Human soul — enters the foetus at the time of birth; Animal soul — enters the embryo at the time of fertilization.

8. Mind is closely related with the skin. So, being subtle in form, it travels the whole body through the skin.
9. Nature of mind is stable and concentrated. But, it becomes unstable due to the influence of different emotions and mental disorders.
10. Mind is an integrated unit of the five elements and acts under the influence of *sattva, raja, tama* — the three cosmic forces. *Sattva* or force of balance is considered as the healthy mental status where as *raja* (force of activation) and *tama* (force of conserve) are considered as conditions which vitiate the mind. Mind, under the influence of these three forces, behaves as follows:

Under influence of	Activities of mind
Sattva — Good mental health	Good sense, wisdom, intelligence, concentration
Raja — Mental disorder	Anger, passion, anxiety, restlessness, joy, jealousy
Tama — Mental disorder	Ignorance, illusion, inappropriate, lethargy, fear, worry, enviness, greediness

The influence of these three forces upon the mind differs among individuals who react differently to a same situation. These three forces are the playmasters of the mind and are responsible for creation of different emotions, thought waves and actions. It may be assumed that the secretion of biochemicals or neurohumours from the endocrine glands or nerve endings is triggered off by the influence of these three forces on the mind under different situations.

1.15 Ayurvedic Concept of the Mind and its Function

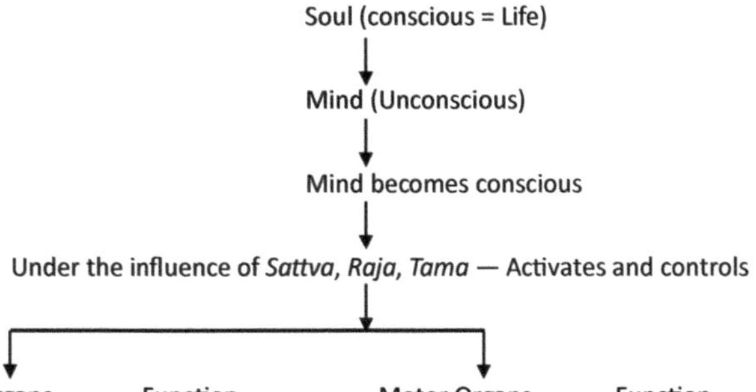

Sense Organs	Function	Motor Organs	Function
Ear (Auditory system)	Hearing	Vocal cord mouth	Speech
Skin	Feeling of touch	Hands	Holding, Movements
Eyes (Organ of vision)	Seeing	Legs	Walking Movements
Tongue (Gustatory system)	Perception of taste	Anus	Excretion
Nose (Olfactory system)	Perception of smell	Genitals	Excretion and sexual functions

References

Acharya, Y.T. (2001). *Ayurved Dipika Commentary of Chakrapani on Charak Samhita*, 5th Edition. Choukhambha Sanskrit Sansthan, Varanasi, India.

Beinfield, H. and Korngold, E. (1991). *Between Heaven and Earth: A Guide to Chinese Medicine*. Ballantine Books, New York.

Bensky, D. and Gamble, A. (1993). *Chinese Herbal Medicine: Materia Medica*. Eastland Press, Seattle, WA.

Cai, G., Chao, G. and Chen, D. (1995). *Advanced Textbook of Traditional Chinese Medicine and Pharmacology*, Vol. 1. New World Press, Beijing.

Encyclopaedia Britannica. (1980). *Encyclopaedia Britannica*, Vol. 6. Churchill-Livingston, London, p. 10.

Filliozat, J. (1964). *The Classical Doctrine of Indian Medicine*. Munshiram Manoharlal Oriental Booksellers and Publishers, Delhi.

Heyn, B. (1987). *Ayurvedic Medicine*. Translated by Louch, D. Thorsons, Wellingsborough.

Lad, V. (1990). *Ayurveda: The Science of Self-Healing*, 2nd Edition. Lotus Press, Twin Lakes, WI.

Maciocia, G. (1989). *The Foundations of Chinese Medicine: A Comprehensive Text for Acupuncturists and Herbalists*. Churchill Livingstone, New York.

O'Brien, K. (2002). Problems and potentials of complementary and alternative medicine. *J. Intern. Med.* **32**, 163–164.

Raina, B.L. (1990). *Health Science in Ancient India*. Commonwealth Publisher, New Delhi.

Ross, J. (1985). *Zang Fu — The Organ Systems of Traditional Chinese Medicine*, 2nd Edition. Churchill Livingston, Edinburgh.

Shastri, A. (1997). *Ayurved Tatwa Sandipika commentary on Sushrut Samhita*, 11th Edition. Choukhambha Sanskrit Sansthan, Varanasi, India.

Takakusu, J. (1956). Observations of medicine in India and China. In: *History of Science in India*. Editorial Enterprises, New Delhi.

Tripathy, B. (1998). *Charak Chandrika Commentary on Charak Samhita*, 5th Edition. Chowkhamba Surbharti Prakashan, Varanasi, India.

Tripathy, B. (2003). *Nirmala Hindi Commentary on Astanga Hridaya*, 1st Edition. Chowkhamba Sanskrit Pratisthan, Delhi, India.

Udupa, K.N. and Singh, R.N. (1978). *Science and Philosophy of Indian Medicine*. Shree Baidyanath Ayurved Bhawan Ltd., Nagpur.

Yin, H.H. and Shuai, H.C. (1992). *Fundamentals of Traditional Chinese Medicine*. Foreign Language Press, Beijing.

Zummer, H.R. (1948). *Hindu Medicine*. Johns Hopkins' Press, Baltimore.

Chapter 2

Ayurveda: Body Structures and Functional Considerations

Debashis Panda

Abstract

Ayurveda is not merely a system of medicine but the science of life. There are two objectives of Ayurveda i.e. first to maintain the good health of healthy individuals and second to cure the disease of the diseased. Panchbhuta (five element) theory and Tridosha (three humour) theory forms the structural and functional basis of Ayurveda and equilibrium in these entities are very essential to achieve the two objectives. In Ayurveda, the concept of seven structural elements is important than internal organs and forms the backbone of Ayurvedic treatment. Ojus i.e. the vital essence of these structural elements is considered as the life energy which is responsible for continuation of Life.

Keywords: Structural Components; Vital Essence; Health Status; Elementary Tissues.

2.1 Structural Landmarks in Ayurveda

Concept of seven structural components is given more importance than internal organs in Ayurveda and forms the backbone of Ayurvedic treatment. In Sanskrit, these are called as *Saptadhātu* where *sapta* means seven and *dhātu* means which that supports the body. These seven structural components not only support the body, but also provide nourishment and are responsible for the growth and maintenance of the body. These can be correlated with the elementary tissues of modern science. They are:

1. *Rasa dhātu* — The blood plasma.
2. *Rakta dhātu* — The formed elements (blood minus plasma) (W.B.C., R.B.C. and platelets).
3. *Mamsa dhātu* — The muscle tissue.
4. *Meda dhātu* — The adipose tissue.
5. *Asthi dhātu* — The bone.
6. *Majjā dhātu* — The red bone marrow.
7. *Sukra dhātu* — The reproductive tissue (semen).

The fundamental concept of Ayurvedic histology is that — each elementary tissue is formed from the previous tissue in descending order. After intestinal digestion, *āhāra rasa* (chyme) is formed. From *āhāra rasa*, *rasa dhātu* or the blood plasma is formed, from blood plasma, formed elements are formed and then muscle tissue, adipose tissue, bone tissue, bone marrow tissue, reproductive tissue are formed one after another from the previous tissues. It usually takes 30 days for the production of reproductive tissue (*sukra dhātu*) from blood plasma (*rasa dhātu*) in the above sequence. However, drugs having special affinity towards reproductive tissue, can produce the reproductive tissue within one day. This is called *prabhāva* in Ayurveda, which means specific potency, hidden action, or unarguable potency of that drug. This principle is similarly applicable to other drugs having special affinity towards producing specific human tissues.

Functions of these seven structural components are:

Rasa dhātu (Plasma)	Nourishment to body cells, creation of formed elements (*rakta dhātu*), refreshes body and mind.
Rakta dhātu (Formed elements)	Provides vitality nourishes and creates muscle tissue.
Mansa dhātu (Muscle tissue)	Strengthens the body and covers body, nourishes and creates adipose tissue.
Meda dhātu (Adipose tissue)	Make oleation of body and secures sturdiness, nourishes and creates bone tissue.

(*Continued*)

(*Continued*)

Asthi dhātu (Bone tissue)	Supports the body, provides the structural architecture to the body. Nourishes and creates bone marrow tissue.
Majjā dhātu (Bone marrow tissue)	Fills the bones, and make oleation of the body. Nourishes and creates reproductive tissue.
Sukra dhātu (Reproductive tissue)	Production of off spring, strengthens the body, responsible for calmness of mind and happiness. The final essence of food and medicine.

The vital essence of all above seven structural components is called as *Ojus*, otherwise known as Life essence. After fertilisation, it appears first as the essence of sperm (*sukra*) and ovum (*sonita*), even before the creation of other seven structural components and circulates throughout the body till the end of Life. It lodges in the heart and circulates in the body along with blood. It is needless to say that death occurs due to complete loss of this vital essence, Ojus. There is some loss of *Ojus* (vital essence) occurs in diseases like diabetes mellitus (*madhumeha*), fever (*jwara*), tuberculosis (*rājayakhmā*), etc., but this loss can be redressed with proper administration of food and medicines. It is slight reddish yellow in colour that resembles the colour of cow's ghee. It is sweet in taste (like honey) and it smells like rice flakes (*lājāgandhi*).

Ojus is of two types, *viz. para ojus* (life energy) and *apara ojus* (supporting energy). *Para ojus* (life energy) resides in the heart, measuring about eight drops and not circulating in nature. *Apara ojus* (supporting life energy) accounts for about 96 grams (*ardhānjali*) and circulates in the whole body through the blood. Normal functions of *ojus* can be perceived as:

(i) Firm and well developed muscular body.
(ii) Unobstructed movement of body parts.
(iii) Clarity of voice and lustrous complexion.
(iv) Normal functioning of external and internal organs.

The most important function of *ojus* is the growth and maintenance of body. It renders the body to overwhelm the aetiological factors of the disease, thus can be ascribed to act as immune system of body. It can be correlated with the immunoglobulins that play a major role in body immune system.

The signs and symptoms of increase, decrease and vitiation of respective structural tissues are described in Ayurvedic classics and from this the

Ayurvedic practitioner assess the patient's condition and treat accordingly. The increased tissue has to be decreased by prescribing medicines which are having opposite qualities to that of the increased *dhātu* or cut out surgically as in case of tumor (*adhimānsa*) or bone growth (*adhyasthi*). The decreased one has to be increased by administering drugs of same qualities. And the vitiated tissue has to be pacified by means of detoxifying techniques (*Panchkarma*) or medicines.

There are seven sub-structural components (*upadhātu*) which are generally by-products of the elementary tissues. These sub-structural components only support the body but do not nourish the body cells. They are:

Sanskrit name	Modern equivalent	By-product of	Function
Stanya	Breast milk	Plasma	Nourishment to baby
ārtava	Menstrual blood and ovum	Plasma	Menstruation and fertilization
Kandarā	Tendons	Blood	Movement of body parts
Sirā	Blood vessels	Blood	Blood circulation
Vasā	Fat tissue	Muscle tissue	Oleation and weight gain
Twak	Skin	Muscle tissue	Covering of body and protection
Snāyu	Nerve tissue	Adipose tissue	Transmission of impulses

Note: Bone, Bone marrow and reproductive tissue have no by-products.

The elementary tissues have seven waste products, which play some roles in maintenance of health status. They are:

Malas in Sanskrit	Comparison	Waste product of	Function
Kapha	Mucus	Plasma	Expulsion in productive cough

(*Continued*)

(*Continued*)

Malas in Sanskrit	Comparison	Waste product of	Function
Pitta	Biles	Blood	Process of digestion (fat emulsification)
Kha mala	Waste secretion of ear, nose, mouth, etc.	Muscle	Prevents environmental pollutants entering body
Sveda	Sweat	Adipose tissue	Maintenance of body temperature
Nakha	Nails	Bone tissue	Protection
Roma	Hair in head and body	Bone tissue	Protection and helps in perspiration
Twak and *Akhi Vit*	Oily secretion of skin and eyes	Bone marrow	Oleation and lustre

Note: Reproductive tissue has no waste products.

The other three principal waste products, formed as end product of metabolism, are urine (*mutra*), faeces (*purisha*) and sweat (*sveda*). Proper evacuation of waste products, not excess nor scanty, is the state of good health and disorder is the diseased state.

2.2 Internal Organs (*Kosthāngas*) in Ayurveda

There are some controversies found among the old classics regarding the number and nomenclature of internal organs. *Charak Samhita*, *Sushruta Samhita* and *Ashtanga Hridaya* are principal treatises of Ayurveda and collectively known as *Brihatrayee* (Major triad). So, we will concentrate on these three treatises to study the descriptions regarding internal organs and evaluate the differences. There are 15 internal organs described in *Charak Samhita*, whereas eight in *Sushruta Samhita* and 11 in *Ashtanga Hridaya*.

The comparison of internal organs, described in these treatises with their modern correlation, is as shown in the following table:

Charak Samhita	*Sushruta Sanshita*	*Ashtanga Hridaya*	Modern correlation
Hridaya	*Hridaya* ✓	✓	Heart
Kloma	*Agnyasaya*	*Kloma*	Pancreas
Yakrit	✓	✓	Liver
Pleeha	×	✓	Spleen
Nābhi	×	✓	Umbilicus
Vrikkak	✓	✓	Kidney
Vasti	×	✓	Urinary bladder
Āmāśaya	✓	×	Stomach
Pakwāsaya	✓	×	Large intestine
Purishdharā	×	×	Epithelial lining of colon
Kshudrāntra	×	×	Small intestine
Sthulāntra	×	*Antra*	Large intestine
Uttara guda	×	×	Rectum
Adhara guda	×	×	Anal canal
Vapāvahana	×	×	Omentum
×	*Phufusa*	✓	Lungs
×	*Unduka*	✓	Ileum, lungs
×	×	*Dimba*	Uterus and ovary

It is quite astonishing that *Charak* doesn't include lungs in the list of internal organs even though he includes less important organs like omentum, rectum, anal canal, etc. in the list. However, *Sushruta* and *Vāgbhatta* include Lungs in their list as an internal organ. The Ayurvedic concept regarding the creation of internal organs in intrauterine life is as follows:

Heart	From excellent essence of blood in combination with the humour *kapha*.
Liver	From excellent portion of blood.
Spleen	From excellent portion of blood.

Lungs	From the froth of blood.
Kidneys	From the essence of blood and fat.
Pancreas	From blood in association with the humour *vāta*.
Ileum and caecum	From the waste product of blood.
Intestines	From the essence of blood and muscles with the help of humour *vāta*.
Tongue	From the essence of blood, muscles and the humour *kapha*.
Testis	From the essence of blood, muscles, fat in association with humour *kapha*.
Eyes	Sclera from kapha, cornea from blood and pupil from both.

2.3 Description of Heart in Ayurveda

In Ayurveda, heart is known as *Hridaya* (in Sanskrit Language), literally which means the organ that receives (blood) gives (blood) and works throughout the day and night. It is formed from the excellent essence of blood in combination with the humour *kapha* (*rakta* + *kapha*). It resembles a lotus bud that is curved and faces downwards. On its left side, lung (left lung) and spleen are situated. The liver and the pancreas are situated on its right side. There is a hollow space inside and it is attached with 24 vessels which carry blood to and from the heart. It houses the soul and mind and so, called as the seat of consciousness. Its functions get diminished, when the person sleeps and it blossoms, when the person gets awakened.

2.3.1 *Āśayas* (*Hollow Organs*) *in Ayurveda*

Literally, *āśaya* means a hollow cavity with space to hold something inside. These are seven *āśayas* as described in Ayurveda.

Name	Modern equivalent	Function
Vātāśaya	Body cavity below umbilical level	Principal site of the humour *vāta*.
Pittāśaya	Body cavity in between umbilicus and Heart	Principal site for the humour *pitta*.

(*Continued*)

(*Continued*)

Name	Modern equivalent	Function
Kaphāśaya	Body cavity above the level of heart	Principal site for the humour *kapha*.
Raktāśaya	Heart	Blood reservoir and helps in blood circulation.
Āmāśaya	Stomach	Reservoir of the undigested food.
Pakwāśaya	Large intestine	Reservoir of the digested food (waste products of digestion).
Mūtrāśaya	Urinary bladder	Reservoir of urine.

There is an extra asaya (hollow organ) in women, i.e. no. 8 (eight) for them, known as *garvāśaya* (the uterus). It is situated in between the *pittāśaya* and *pakwāśaya*.

2.3.2 *Kalā* (*Membranes*)

When the moisture present in between the elementary tissues (*dhātu*) and hollow space (*āśaya*) gets processed by their own heat, some membrane-like structures known as *kalā* are created. They resemble the stem bark of trees covering the heartwood. They are again seven in number:

1. *Mānsadharā kalā*: It is the first variety of membrane present in muscles, which holds the veins, ligaments, nerves and arteries inside the muscles. Similar to the stalks and stems of lotus plant coming out of ground, these vessels and nerves pervade in the muscles in different directions.
2. *Raktadharā kalā*: This second variety of membrane is present inside the muscles, particularly in veins, spleen and liver, which contains blood. It can be correlated with inner epithelial linings of vessels. When there is a cut in muscles, bleeding occurs just as milk oozes when there is a cut in milky tree.
3. *Medodharā kalā*: This third variety of membrane holds the fat or adipose tissue. Fat, found in long stout bones, is called as bone marrow (yellowish), however, red bone marrow (*sarakta meda*) is found in other smaller bones. Fat as pure form of muscles is found particularly inside the abdomen.

4. *Slesmadharā kalā*: It is a greasy substance (synovial fluid), found in all joints inside the synovial membrane that helps in lubrication of joints just as oil is needed for the proper functioning of wheels.
5. *Purishdharā kalā*: It is present inside the small intestine and large intestine (epithelial inner linings of intestine). At the site of caecum (*unduka*), it separates the faecal matter from the digested food.
6. *Pittadharā kalā*: It is situated in between the stomach (*Āmāśaya*) and intestine (*pakwāśaya*). It holds the undigested food for a while to digest it properly by the heat of *pitta* (*agnāśaya*) and then allows the digested food to move further. It is also called as *grahanī* (duodenum). If it gets vitiated, it can't digest the food and allows the undigested food to move downward, causing a disease known as *Grahanīdosha* (irritable bowel syndrome).
7. *Sukradharā kalā*: This seventh membrane holds the semen and pervades the entire body. However, the ejaculatory membrane (passage) is present two fingers (breadth) away from the opening of urinary bladder on the right side connecting with the urethra.

2.3.3 *Bones (Asthi)*

There are five types of bones present in our body. They are:

Bone type	Meaning	Site
Kapāla	Flat bones	Hip bone, scapula, patella, palate temporal bones, skull.
Ruchaka	Peg like	Teeth.
Taruna	Tender bones or cartilage	Present in nose, ears, throat and eye sockets.
Valaya	Curved or ring like	Present in feet, hands, back and abdomen (tarsal, carpal bone and vertebrae).
Nalak	Long bones	Rest bones (like humerus, radius, ulna, femur, tibia, fibula, ribs, etc.)

Bones are 300 in number, out of which 120 are present in the extremities, 117 in the trunk and the rest 63 in the head and neck region.

2.3.4 *Joints* (*Sandhi*)

Primarily, the joints are of two types *viz.* mobile (*chestāvanta*) and immobile (*sthira*). Again, the joints are divided into eight groups. The nature and location of joints are as follows:

Joint type	Modern correlation	Location
Kora	Hinge joint	Fingers, ankles, knees, wrists and elbows
Udukhal	Ball and socket joint	Axillae (shoulder joint, groins (hip joint), roots of teeth
Sāmudga	Covering joints or sealed joints	Shoulder, rectum, pelvis, buttocks
Pratara	Spear shaped or rounded	Neck and vertebral column
Tunnasevani	Suturing joints	Flat bone of head and pelvis
Vāyasatunda	Crow's beak shaped joint	Both sides of lower jaw (mandibular joints)
Mandal	Circular joints	Throat, eyes, cardiac region and trachea
Sankhāvarta	Spiral shaped	Internal ear and sphenoidal region

Total number of joints in the body is 210, out of which 68 joints are present in the extremities, 59 in the trunk and 83 in the head and neck region.

2.3.5 *Muscle* (*Mānsapeśī*)

Muscles are 500 in number, out of which 400 are found in the extremities, 66 in the trunk and rest 34 in the head and neck. Additional 20 muscles are found in females. Five muscles are present in each breast, four in vagina and six in uterus.

2.3.6 *Vein (Sirā)*

Veins are 700 in number, out of which 400 are present in the extremities (100 in each), 136 in the trunk and rest 164 in the head and neck region. Venous puncture (*sirā vedha*) or bloodletting is a famous and effective surgical treatment in Ayurveda. Site of venous puncture and the methodology is vividly described in *Sushruta Samhita.* Out of 700 veins, 98 veins should not be punctured (*avedhya sirā*) and the surgeon should be cautious while performing surgery around these veins. Sixteen unpuncturable veins are located in the extremities, and 32 in the trunk and 50 in the head and neck region.

2.3.7 *Main Arteries (Mūla Dhamanī)*

Main arteries are 24 in number, out of them 10 spread upwards, 10 downwards and four sideways. Each artery moving upward and downward again divided into three branches, thus making 60 (30 + 30) arteries. Arteries moving sideways have innumerable branches.

2.3.8 *Ligaments (Snāyu)*

Ligaments are 900 in number, out of which 600 are present in the extremities (150 in each extremity), 230 in the trunk, 34 in head and 36 in neck region. Ligaments are of four types.

1. *Pratānavati* — flat and thin — found in extremities and joints.
2. *Vritta* — rounded — big tendons.
3. *Sushira* — porous — found in urinary bladder, stomach and intestines.
4. *Prithū* — thick — found in flanks, back, chest, neck and head.

2.3.9 *Big Tendons (Kandarā)*

Big tendons are 16 in number, out of which eight are found in the extremities (two each), four in the back and the rest four in the neck.

2.3.10 *Net-like Structures* (*Jāla*)

Net-like structures comprise muscles, veins, ligaments and nerves intertwined altogether. They are 16 in number, eight in extremities, four in neck and four in back.

2.3.11 *Brush Like Structure* (*Kūrca*)

These are six in number, one in each hand and feet, one in neck and one in penis.

2.3.12 *Rope of Muscles* (*Rajju*)

These are four in number, situated on either side of the vertebral column (two on each side), for binding the muscles.

2.3.13 *Sutures* (*Sīvanī*)

Sutures are seven in number, out of which five are present in the brain, and one each in tongue and penis.

2.3.14 *Confluence of Bones* (*Sanghāta*)

Confluence of bones are 14, and these are two ankle joints, two knee joints, two hip joints, two wrist joints, two elbow joints, two shoulder joints, one pelvic joint and one in the head.

2.4 Transporting Channels (*srotas*) in Ayurveda

Transporting channels (*srotas*) are hollow pipe-like structures in the human body, through which body fluids, nutrients, food, oxygen, water or waste products are transported from one place to another. Literally, the word *srotas* in Sanskrit means the structures in which oozing or trickling of fluids is possible. This means *srotas* are semi-permeable in nature and may encompass the blood vessels, G.I.T. and other hollow pipe-like (tubular) structures of body. They may be macroscopic (*sthula*) or microscopic (*Anu*) in appearance, their branches pervade to every part of the body like a creeper with many branches pervading to every part of the body and supplying nutrients for the nourishment of homologous body tissues.

The colour of the *srotas* (transporting channel) is dependent on the substance that flows inside it. Unless and until the flow of the nutrients or body fluids is disturbed, there would be continuation of good health. There are 13 transporting channels described in *Charak Samhita*, each of which has two distinct roots i.e. the controlling centres. The first three channels (*prānavaha*, *udakavaha*, *annavaha*) are connected with external environment and bring oxygen (breathing), water and food into the body for maintenance of life. The last three channels (*mūtravaha*, *purishvaha* and *svedavaha*) expel out the body excreta i.e. the waste products of metabolism. The rest of the seven channels transport the seven structural components of the body (*sapta dhātus*), supply the excellent product of digestion i.e. nutrients to augment respective structural homologues. These seven channels are responsible for nourishment of body cells and tissues. Nevertheless, every channel is important, and their proper functioning is to be maintained for achieving good health. The transporting channels are:

Channels	Correlation	Site of origin (roots)
Vitality (O_2) transporting	Respiratory system	Lungs, heart and blood vessels
Water transporting	Mouth, oesophagus, stomach	Palate, pancreas
Food transporting	G.I.T.	Stomach, G.I.T.
Plasma transporting	Circulatory system	Heart, blood vessels
Formed element transporting	Circulatory system	Liver, spleen
Muscles tissue transporting	Circulatory system	Ligaments, skin
Adipose tissue transporting	Circulatory system	Kidney, omentum
Bone tissue transporting	Circulatory system	Adipose tissue, pelvis
Marrow tissue transporting	Circulatory system	Bone, joints
Reproductive tissue transporting	Reproductive system	Testis, urethra
Urine transporting	Urinary system	Kidney, urinary bladder

(*Continued*)

(*Continued*)

Channels	Correlation	Site of origin (roots)
Faeces transporting	Large intestine and anus	Sigmoid colon, rectum
Sweat transporting	Perspiration	Adipose tissue, hair follicles

Here, it is assumed that the transporting channel from 4 to 09 is one and the same i.e. the circulatory system. Though, circulatory system serves as a common conduit for the transportation of body tissue (no. 7), Ayurvedic considers each channel as separate conduit system. They are concerned about the presence of nutrients, which will augment respective homologous body tissues only, not others. For example, proteins or nitrogenous compounds (amino acids) nourish muscle tissues, iron nourishes blood tissue, fatty acid and glycerol replenish adipose tissue, calcium, magnesium nourish bone tissue, etc. Each transporting channel has separate two distinct roots i.e. the controlling centres. Each conduit system is separate from the other and has its own importance, injury to these channels causes giddiness, delusion, tremors, delirium, pain, flatulence, indigestion, loss of appetite, thirst, vomiting, fever, severe bleeding, urinary dysfunction, constipation diarrhoea and even death. When there is a foreign body lodged inside, it should be removed first and then treated as a fresh wound. Due to unhealthy dietary intake and behavioural practice, these channels get vitiated and cause diseases. Vitiation of channels is of four types *viz.* (1) excess functioning (*atipravritti*), (2) obstruction or hypo-activity (*saṅga*), (3) tumours or swelling (*sirāgranthi*), (4) movement in opposite or wrong direction (*vimārga gamana*). Albeit, the cause of vitiation is different for each channel and so are the signs and symptoms. The cause of vitiation, signs and symptoms and treatment of all the channels are depicted below.

(1) *Prānavaha Srotas* (Respiratory System)

Cause of vitiation — loss of body tissues, intake of dry foods, doing exercise in a state of hunger or thirst, suppression of natural urges and other abnormal activities.

Signs and symptoms — continuous, excess or obstructed respiration. Expiration associated with pain and sound, giddiness, delusion.

Treatment — same as asthma (*swāsh*) or dyspnoea (*swashkasta*).

(2) *Udakavaha Srotas* (Water Transporting Channel)
Cause of vitiation — consumption of excess alcohol, hot and dry foods, astringent foods, indigestion of food, suppression of thirst, fear.
Signs and symptoms — excessive thirst, dryness of mouth, dryness and dysfunction of pancreas, ringing in ear (tinnitus), unconsciousness.
Treatment — appropriate water intake, administering moisture containing herbs and treatment of thirst.

(3) *Annavaha Srotas* (Food Transporting Channel)
Cause of vitiation — due to imbalanced or weak digestive fire (enzymes), intake of food before digestion of previous meal, intake of excess food, uncooked food, consumption of incompatible foods together, excess fasting, unwholesome food, irregular diet habit.
Signs and symptoms — indigestion, anorexia, loss of appetite, vomiting, diarrhoea, flatulence, headache.
Treatment — stomachics and digestives, therapeutic purgation.

(4) *Rasavaha Srotas* (Plasma Transporting Channel)
Cause of vitiation — indigestion, less intake of nutrients, anxiety, worry, intake of heavy, cold and too oily food.
Signs and symptoms — fever, body ache, palpitation, anaemia, lean body, impotence, low digestive fire.
Treatment — easy digestible nutritive diet, occasional fasting, intake of digestives (improve digestion).

(5) *Raktavaha Srotas* (Formed Element Transporting Channel)
Cause of vitiation — more spicy, hot, oily and irritant foods, excess exposure to heat and sun.
Signs and symptoms — skin disease, erysipelas, bleeding disorder, bleeding from the external openings, splenomegaly, Jaundice, Leukoderma, abscess, menorrhagia, metrorrhagia.
Treatment — therapeutic purgation, haemostatic and blood purifier drugs, mild fasting, bloodletting.

(6) *Māṅsavaha Srotas* (Muscle Tissue Transporting Channel)
Cause of vitiation — over consumption of meat, more intake of sweet, heavy, cold things, sleeping immediately after lunch.
Signs and symptoms — tumour, uneven growth, scrofula, goitre.
Treatment — therapeutic vomiting and purgation, surgery, cauterization (*agnikarma*), caustics application (*ksāra karma*)*.

**Ksāra Karma* is one of the most important para surgical procedures of Ayurveda. *Ksāra* means the concentrated salts or alkali substances found in herbs. It is prepared by evaporating the water mixed up with the ashes of specific alkali herbs. Sometimes, some minerals are added to get a strong *ksāra* or caustics. When applied locally, *ksāra* is capable of carrying out functions like incision, excision and scraping with simultaneous healing.

(7) *Medovaha Srotas* (Adipose Tissue Transporting Channel)
Cause of vitiation — excess consumption of fatty foods and lack of physical activities, excess sleep, excess intake of alcohols.
Signs and symptoms — prodromal signs and symptoms of diabetes mellitus (unwilling to work (lethargic)), burning sensation in hands and feet, dryness of throat and palate, heaviness of body parts, looseness of body, profuse sweating and foul smelling of body), obesity, debilitated and lean body (emaciation).
Treatment — treatment for diabetes (*madhumeha*), obesity (*sthaulya*) and other diseases as they develop.

(8) *Asthivaha Srotas* (Bone Tissue Transporting Channels)
Cause of vitiation — intake of dry, light, cold food, over consumption of pungent, bitter and astringent food, sedentary life style.
Signs and symptoms — pain in bones, brittleness of bones, extra bone growth, diseases of hair and beard (greying and falling) diseases of nails.
Treatment — therapeutic enema, administration of drugs with bitter taste processed with milk and butter.

(9) *Majjāvaha Srotas* (Marrow Tissue Transporting Channels)
Cause of vitiation — traumatic injury (crushing), compression of bone marrow, taking food devoid of fat, incompatible foods taken together.
Signs and symptoms — giddiness, unconsciousness, pain in small joints, darkness in front of eyes (*tamodarsana*).
Treatment — food and medicine having sweet and bitter taste, proper elimination of body toxins in appropriate season, proper exercise and controlled sexual activity.

(10) *Sukravaha Srotas* (Reproductive Tissue Transporting Channel)
Cause of vitiation — excess and inappropriate sexual act, traumatic injury by surgical instrument, caustics and cauterisation instruments, suppression of sexual urges.

Signs and symptoms — impotence, unpleasurable sexual act, no conception or if conception occurs, results in abortion.
Treatment — food and medicine with sweet and bitter taste processed in milk and butter, therapeutic purificatory procedures (vomiting and purgation), proper exercise and controlled sexual activity.

(11) *Mūtravaha Srotas* (Urine Transporting Channels)
Cause of vitiation — suppression of urinary urge while taking food and water or having sexual intercourse by suppressing the urge to urinate, external injury to debilitated person.
Signs and symptoms — urinary dysfunction, painful burning micturition, scanty, more viscous urination.
Treatment — diuretic herbs, excess intake of water, treatments as described in urinary dysfunction.

(12) *Purishvaha Srotas* (Faeces Transporting Channels)
Cause of vitiation — dry foods, suppression of urge to defecate, poor digestive fire, emaciated person, over-eating in indigestion.
Signs and symptoms — constipation, painful defecation, occasional diarrhoea.
Treatment — increase the digestive power, increase the appetite, and other treatment as described for diarrhoea.

(13) *Svedavaha Srotas* (Sweat Transporting Channels)
Cause of vitiation — excessive exercise, exposure to cold soon after heat exposure and *vice versa*, anger, fear, grief.
Signs and symptoms — profuse sweating or absence of sweating, burning sensation.
Treatment — sudorifics, treatment as described for fever.

In addition to above, there are two extra channels found in females. They are menstrual blood transporting channels (*ārtavavaha srotas*) and breast milk transporting channels (*stanyavaha srotas*). The menstrual blood transporting channel has two roots *viz.* uterus and endometrium (*ārtavavahi dhamanīs*). Signs and symptoms of vitiation of this channel are infertility, dyspareunia and amenorrhoea. Drugs of hot nature are administered after proper purification to correct this channel. Breast milk transporting channel or lactation system also has two roots i.e. breasts and lactation ducts (*stanyavahi dhamanis*). Signs and symptoms of vitiation of this channel are tender breasts, diminished breast milk and impure breast milk. Causes may be external trauma, anxiety, fear, more workload, consumption of dry, rough, hot and more spicy foods. Galactogogues and breast milk purifier herbs along with the herbs that increase blood plasma (*rasa dhātu*) are to be administered for its treatment.

Though not included among 13 transporting channels, *manovaha srotas* (psychological channels) cannot be ignored and it is described by many ancient authors in the context of mind. These are the channels that carry cyclic impulses and are principally responsible for memory i.e. intellect or power of acquisition (*dhi*), power of retention (*dhruti*) and power of recollection (*smruti*). There are no roots attributed to these psychological channels, but the brain and heart can be considered as their roots. The mind is inherently related (*samavāya sambandha*) with the skin and thus moves everywhere through it. So, the skin acts as a conduit system for the mind, where mind is separate from memory. Even so, they are complementary to each other and influence each other's action. *Manovaha srotas* (psychological channels) deals with both these aspects. It is vitiated due to behavioral defective attitudes and bad conducts and resulted in a series of mental disorders. These conditions can be treated with the brain tonics (*medhya rasāyana*) and *sirodhārā* (a treatment procedure, in which herbal decoction, oils or milk is poured over the forehead in a continuous stream for a definite period). Non-material treatment includes *prānāyāma* (breath holding technique) and *dhyāna* (meditation), both are two sub-stages of Yoga.

2.4.1 *The Skin (Tvak)*

The skin is often considered as the largest organ of the human body because of its largest surface area. Furthermore, it accounts for about 15% of total body weight, which is much larger than any of the internal organ. In Ayurveda, the skin is regarded as one of the sense organs and known as *sparśanendriya* (tactile sensory organ). It is composed of all the five elements, however, air is predominant among them. It also acts as a chief site for the humour *vata*. At the same time, it also serves as the dwelling of *bhrājaka pitta* (one sub-type of the humour *pitta*, which regulates body temperature and skin pigmentation). The skin is associated with the perception of touch along with sensations of pain, heat, cold, rough, smooth, etc. The most important aspect of skin in Ayurveda is its inherent relationship (*samavāya sambandha*) with mind. Mind travels through the skin and gets connected with different body parts. It also acts as an important route of drug administration as it absorbs the medicinal properties of locally applied medicinal herbs, oils, smearings, ointments, etc.

Carma is synonymous with the word *tvak* (skin), which literally means "a shield" and signifies the protective action of skin. The skin also excretes the sweat (*sveda*), which is considered as a waste product in Ayurveda.

Sushruta, the father of surgery, described seven layers of skin in his ancient book *Sushruta Samhita*, whereas *Charak* described six layers of skin. The Ayurvedic view of creation of skin in embryonic stage is very interesting. All the ancient scholars of Ayurveda unanimously described the formation of skin from the metabolism of blood after the formation of zygote as similar to the formation of cream layer on the surface of boiling milk. Since skin is formed from blood, brightness of skin indicates the purity of blood and rough, dry, dull skin indicates impure blood. *Charak* described skin as one of the sub-structural components (*upadhātu*) of body, which is produced from the muscle tissue. The seven layers of skin can be correlated with five layers of epidermis, dermis and sub-cutis, which signifies ancient Indian Medical Science to be very scientific.

Skin layers in Ayurveda	Modern comparison	Breadth of skin layer as described in Ayurveda
Avabhāsinī	Stratum corneum	1/18th part of a rice grain (*Vrihī*)
Lohitā	Stratum lucidum	1/16th part of a rice grain
Śvetā	Stratum granulosum	1/12th part of a rice grain
Tāmrā	Stratum spinosum	1/8th part of a rice grain
Vedinī	Stratum germinativum/ basale	1/5th part of rice grain

(*Continued*)

(*Continued*)

Skin layers in Ayurveda	Modern comparison	Breadth of skin layer as described in Ayurveda
Rohinī	Dermis	Same as a rice grain
Mānsadharā	Sub-cutis	Double the breadth of a rice grain

Note: Every successive layer is thicker than the previous one.

2.4.2 *Individual Description of Seven Skin Layers*

Avabhāsinī — It is the outermost and thinnest layer of skin. This layer is responsible for skin lustre and five different shades (*chāya*) and seven reflections (*prabhā*). It has the ability to retain water and helps in the moisturisation of the skin. Keeping in view this function, *Charak* has named this layer as *udakadharā* (*udaka* means water and *dharā* means to hold). This is similar to the function of stratum corneum, which hydrates the skin by absorbing water and preventing water evaporation. When this layer gets vitiated, diseases like dandruff, fungal infection, acne, pimples occur.

Lohitā — The second layer of skin is called *lohitā* (red) because of its redness in colour. According to *Charak*, it holds the blood (*asrikdharā*). The diseases which affect this layer are moles (*tilakalaka*), dark circles (*nyachha*), black pigmentation (*vyanga*), etc.

Śvetā — This third layer is whitish in colour. This is the site for diseases like eczema (*charmadala*), allergic rashes (*ajagallikā*) and big moles (*masaka*).

Tāmrā — This fourth layer is copper in colour and serves as the site for the disease like Leukoderma, and other skin diseases. However, diseases like albinism, melanoma and basal cell carcinoma are found in stratum germinativum (basale) in the modern point of view.

Vedinī — This fifth layer is meant for the pain sensation. Diseases like leprosy (*kustha*), erysipelas, herpes (*visarpa*) and other skin diseases affect this layer.

Rohinī — This sixth layer grows the skin and replenishes the other layers of skin. When this layer gets vitiated, diseases like tumour (*arbuda*), knot-like structures (*granthi*), glandular swelling around neck (*galaganda*) and other swelling disorders occur.

However, in the modern point of view, skin cell replenishing function is attributed to stratum germinativum, which lies at the base of epidermis and immediately above dermis. Again, the pain sensation quality is attributed to the dermis layer. Many nerve endings are present in the dermis that provide the sense of touch, pain, heat and cold.

Charak has described six layers of skin and given more importance to the sixth layer. He describes this layer as the supporter of life (*prānadharā*) because of the presence of nerve endings and blood vessels in it. Incision or cutting of this layer causes severe pain, darkness in front of eyes (*tama-pravesh*) and unconsciousness. He also advocates one incurable disease, namely, *arunshi* in this layer, which is deep rooted and reddish-black in colour. This could be correlated with melanoma or basal cell carcinoma.

Mānsadharā: This is the seventh and inner most layer of skin as described by *Sushruta*. It holds the muscles, which means it covers the muscles underlying this layer, and hence the name *mānsadharā* (*mānsa* — muscles and *dharā* — to hold). It can be correlated with the sub cutis layer. Diseases like piles (*arsa*), fistula (*bhagandara*) and abscess (*vidradhi*) occur in these layers.

2.4.3 *The Science of Vital Points* (*Marma Vijnāna*)

The science of vital points is considered half of the subject surgery in Ayurveda. Literally, the word *Marma* in Sanskrit means "that kills" or "which gives unbearable pain". This means injury to these points causes death or serious consequences including morbidity and severe pain. These vulnerable or sensitive points are meant to be protected cautiously during surgery. These vital points play an important role in Indian martial arts and need to be protected against injury in the battlefield. In this connection, *marmas* (vital points) are considered as "seats of life" (*prānāyātana*) in Ayurveda. Therapeutically, these vital points can be manipulated with pressure (or massage) or needles (marmapuncture, practised in South India and Sri Lanka) to influence the physiological and pathological states. The *marma* points (vital points) are analogous with the acupoints of Traditional Chinese Medicines (TCMs) but not exactly the same. Acupoints are defined as "holes of deliverance" or "transportation holes", that are present on meridians (conduits) or meeting points of different meridians. Therapeutically, these acupoints are punctured with needles to alter the flow of *Qi* and this treatment modality is known as Acupuncture, which is an important branch of Chinese medicine. On the other hand, *marmas* are meeting point of veins, arteries, tendons, muscles, bones and joints in the body. These are also related to the transporting channels (*srotas*), nervous system (*nādi* and *shat chakras*) and concept of three humours. There are 107 *marmas* (vital points) found in Ayurveda, whereas 295 acupoints are described in *Nei Jing*, one of the famous treatise in Chinese medicine. However, modern acupuncturists recognise up to more than 1,000 acupoints. *Marmas* in Ayurveda vary in their sizes from 1/2 of the breadth of a finger to the size of a palm. In contrast, acupoints are smaller in size and more superficial (Chattopadhyaya, 1977).

In short, *marmas* can be summarised as:

1. The seat of life (*prānāyātana*).
2. Where muscles, veins, tendons, nerves, bones and joints meet.
3. Presence of three humours (*vāta, pitta, kapha*).
4. Presence of three gunas (*sattva, raja, tama*).
5. Energy points, that can be stimulated by therapeutic intervention.

2.5 Classification of Marmas

Marmas (vital points) are classified mainly in four ways *viz.* according to their dominant physical constituent or their vulnerability to injury or their dimension or their site. On the basis of their dominant physical constituent, they are classified into five groups (Dharmalingam *et al.*, 1991). They are:

(i) *Sadya Prāṇahara* — Immediate death or death within seven days.
(ii) *Kālāntara Prāṇahara* — Death within 30 days after the exposure to trauma or injury.
(iii) *Vaikalyakara* — It creates morbidity or deformity.
(iv) *Vishalyaghna* — Death occurs when the lodged foreign body is removed. However, life continues as long as the foreign body remains lodged at the injury site (*marma* site).
(v) *Rujākara* — Injury causes severe pain at the *marma* site.

Marmas predominantly have one or two elements from the five-element group and so differ in their vulnerability depending upon the susceptibility and nature of the elements.

Marma	Predominant elements	Number
Sadya Prāṇahara	Fire	19
Kālāntara Prāṇahara	Fire + Water	33
Vaikalyakara	Water	44
Vishalyaghna	Air	03
Rujākara	Air + Fire	08
	Total	107

Moreover, the *marmas* are divided by their dimensions or size. They vary in their size starting from 1/2 of the breadth of a finger (own finger) to the size of a palm (own palm). Number of *marmas* (vital points) measuring 1/2 of the breath of a finger is 56, measuring one finger is 14, measuring two fingers is 4, measuring three fingers is also four, and those measuring about the size of a palm is 29.

There are 44 *marmas* (vital points) found in the extremities, 11 in each one. Twelve *marmas* are found on the anterior side of the trunk and 14 are found on the posterior side. The rest, 37 *marmas*, are present in the head and neck region.

2.5.1 *Individual Description of Marmas*

There are 11 *marmas* present in each extremity. They are:

(1) *Kshipra Marma* — In the leg, it is situated in between the big toe and first toe, and similarly in between the thumb and the index finger in the hand. Injury to this vital point leads to death from convulsion. Though it is considered as *kālāntara prāṇahara marma* (death within one month), sometimes instantaneous death occurs due to severe injury to this *marma*. It is a ligament and nerve-based *marma* (*snāyu marma*) and measures about 1/2 of breadth of finger.

(2) *Tala hridaya Marma* — This vital point is situated in the middle of the sole or palm in a straight line drawn from the root of middle toe or middle finger. Injury to this point leads to death from severe pain. It is a muscle-based *marma* (*mānsa marma*) and death occurs within one

month after the injury. Even when one of the legs or hands is cut down, the person survives, but a person never survives when there is severe injury to this vital spot. So, in case of severe injury to this vital spot, it is advisable to amputate the limb to save the life. The dimension of this spot is about 1/2 of breadth of a finger.

(3) *Kūrca Marma* — It is situated on the dorsal side of the foot or palm above *kshipra marma*, two-finger width on either side. Injury to this *marma* results in shivering and bending of the foot or hand. The patient is unable to rotate and move his foot or hand. It is a nerve-based *marma* and measures about the size of a palm.

(4) *Kūrcaśira Marma* — It is situated just below the ankle joint or wrist joint, measuring about one finger in breadth. Injury to this spot produces pain and swelling. It is a nerve-based *marma.*

(5) *Gulpha Marma* — It is present inside the ankle joint. *Manibandha marma* is present inside the wrist joint. Both these vital spots measure about two fingers in (breadth) dimension and are structurally joint-based *marmas* (*sandhi marma*). Injury to these points causes pain, stiffness and deformity (maimedness).

(6) *Indravasti Marma* — It is situated at the centre of the leg (may be in calf muscle) posterior side, twelve fingers above the heel on a straight line, It measures about 1/2 of the finger breadth. Injury to this vital spot causes excessive haemorrhage leading to death within 30 days (*Kālāntara prānahara*). It is a muscle-based *marma. Indravasti marma* is also found in the middle of fore arm.

(7) *Janu Marma* — It is situated in the knee joint. It is a joint-based *marma*, measuring about three fingers in length and belongs to the *vaikalyakara* group i.e. creates deformity after exposure to injury. Injury to *Janu marma* creates lameness of the patient. Similar to *janu marma* is *kurpara marma* in hands inside the elbow joint, which creates dangling of the hand after exposure to an injury.

(8) *Āni Marma* — It is situated at the point three fingers above to knee joint or elbow joint. It is a ligament (or nerve)-based *marma*, measuring about 1/2 of the breadth of finger and belongs to the *vaikalyakara* group that creates deformity. Injury to this spot creates swelling and paralysis of the respective limb.

(9) *Urvī Marma* — It is situated at the middle of thigh or arm. It is one type of vessel-based *marma*, measuring about one finger in

dimension and belongs to the *vaikalyakara* group that creates deformity. Injury to this *marma* causes haemorrhage leading to atrophy of the limb.

(10) *Lohitāksha Marma* — It is situated above the *urvī marma* but below the hip joint at the root of the thigh. It is a vessel-based *marma*, measuring about 1/2 of the finger in size and belongs to the *vaikalya-kara* group, that creates deformity. Injury to this *marma* causes blood loss leading to hemiplegia. At the same point, this *marma* is present in the arms with similar consequences.

(11) *Vitapa Marma* — It is situated in between the scrotum and inguinal region. It is a nerve (or ligament)-based *marma*, measuring about one finger in dimension and belongs to *vaikalyakara* group. Injury to *vitapa marma* results in impotence and deficiency of semen. *Kakshadhara marma* is the counterpart of *vitapa marma*, present in between axilla and chest region. An injury to *kakshadhara marma* creates paralysis of the hand (hemiplegia).

These are the 11 vital points present in each limb, in this way 44 vital points in the extremities have been described.

2.5.2 *Marmas of Anterior Side of Trunk*

There are 12 vital spots (*marmas*) present in the anterior side of the trunk. They are:

(1) *Guda Marma* — The rectum is called as *guda marma*, which is attached to large intestine and serves as the passage for faeces and flatus. It is one type of muscle-based *marma*, measuring about the size of own palm (four-finger) and belongs to *sadya prāṇahara* group that causes sudden death.

(2) *Vasti Marma* — The urinary bladder is considered as *vasti marma* which is present inside the pelvis and is made up of less muscle and blood. It is a ligament-based *marma*, measuring about the size of own palm and belongs to *sadya prāṅahara* group that causes immediate death within 24 hours or 7 days after injury.

(3) *Nābhi Marma* — Umbilicus is considered as *nābhi marma*, and serves as the root of all the vessels. It is present in between stomach (*āmāśaya*)

and sigmoid colon (*pakvāśaya*). It is a vessel-based *marma*, measuring about the size of own palm and belongs to *sadya prāṇahara* group i.e. immediate death or death within 7 days.

(4) *Hridaya Marma* — The heart is known as *hridaya marma* and is the site for three qualities *sattva*, *raja* and *tama*. It is a vessel-based *marma*, measuring about the size of own palm and belongs to *sadya prāṇahara* group that causes immediate death.

(5) *Stana mūla Marma* — This *marma* is situated two fingers below the breasts on both sides. It is vessel-based *marma*, measuring about one finger and belongs to *kālāntara prāṇahara* group i.e. death within a month. Injury to this *marma* causes accumulation of mucus in the chest leading to death due to cough and dyspnoea within one month. They are two in number, one each on either side.

(6) *Stanarohita Marma* — It is situated two fingers above the nipple on both sides and are two in number. It is a muscle-based *marma*, measuring about 1/2 of the finger breadth and belongs to *kālāntara prāṇahara* group. Injury to this *marma* causes accumulation of blood inside chest leading to death due to cough and dyspnoea within one month.

(7) *Apalāpa Marma* — It is situated below the shoulder joint on the upper corner of the chest. This is vessel-based *marma*, measuring about 1/2 of the finger breadth and belongs to *kālāntara prāṇahara* group. Injury to this *marma* causes accumulation of pus resulting from blood leading to death within one month. These are also two in number, on either side of the chest.

(8) *Apastambha Marma* — The two bronchus are considered as *apastambha marmas* carrying air to the lungs. These are two in number and situated on either side of trachea. These are vessel-based *marmas* measuring about 1/2 of the finger breadth and belongs to *kālāntara prānahara* group. Injury to these *marmas* causes accumulation of air inside the chest leading to death due to cough and dyspnoea within one month.

2.5.3 *Marmas of Posterior Side of Trunk*

There are 14 vital spots (*marmas*) present on the posterior side of the trunk. They are:

(1) *Katikataruna Marma* — The hip bone is considered as *katikataruna marma*, situated on either side of the vertebral column (ear shaped bones of the pelvis). It is a bone-based *marma*, measuring about 1/2 of the finger breadth (may be one particular point on the hip bone) and belongs to *kālāntara prāṇahara* group. Injury to this point causes blood loss, pallor, emaciation leading to death within one month.

(2) *Kukundara Marma* — It is present inside the sacroilliac joint on both sides of the vertebral column, slightly below the waist. It is a joint-based *marma*, measuring about 1/2 of the finger breadth and belongs to *vaikalyakara* group. Injury to this point causes loss of sensation and movement in the lower parts of the body.

(3) *Nitamba Marma* — It is present on the sacral ala or sacral foramina and attached inside to the muscles of the waist. It is a bone-based *marma*, measuring about 1/2 of the finger breadth and belongs to the *kālāntara prāṇahara* group. Injury to this point causes atrophy and weakness in the lower part of the body leading to death within one month.

(4) *Parśvasandhi Marma* — It is situated at the loin, at the lower end of the flanks, sidewards and upwards. This is a vessel-based *marma*, measuring about 1/2 of the finger breadth and belongs to the *kālāntara prāṇahara* group. Injury to this point causes accumulation of blood in the abdomen leading to death within one month.

(5) *Brihati Marma* — It is situated on the posterior side in a straight line with *stanamula marma* (root of the breast) on either side of the vertebral column. This is a vessel-based *marma*, measuring about 1/2 of the breadth of a finger and belongs to *kālāntara prāṇahara* group, i.e. death within one month. Injury to this site causes excessive haemorrhage leading to death.

(6) *Amsaphalaka Marma* — It is present on the scapula bone in both sides. It is a bone based *marma*, measuring about 1/2 of the finger breadth and belongs to the *vaikalyakara group*, that creates deformity. Injury to this point causes atrophy of the arms leading to loss of tactile sensation.

(7) *Amsa Marma* — It is situated in between the neck and head of the arms, connecting the shoulder with the nape of the neck. It is a ligament-based *marma* (*snāyu marma*), measuring about 1/2 of the finger breadth and belongs to *vaikalyakara* group, that creates deformity. Injury to this point causes stiffness in the arms.

All the vital points on posterior side are two in number, present on either side of the vertebral column. So, a total of 14 vital points are present in the posterior side of the trunk.

2.5.4 *Marmas of Neck and Head Region (Jatrurdhvagata Marmas)*

(1) *Nilā* and *Manyā* — These are four in number, two each on either side of the larynx. These are vessel-based *marmas*, measuring about four fingers length and belongs to *vaikalyakara* group i.e. creates deformity. Injury to these vital points causes dumbness, speech disorder and loss of taste perception.

(2) *Sirā Mātrukā Marma* — These are eight in number, four each on either side of the neck. These are vessel-based *marmas*, measuring about four fingers length and belongs to *sadya prāṇahara* group, i.e. immediate death following injury.

(3) *Krikātikā* — These are two in number, present at the junction point of head and neck. These may be correlated with the transverse processes of the arch of atlas. These are joint-based *marmas*, measuring about 1/2 of the finger breadth and belongs to the *vaikalyakara* group that creates deformity. Injury to this point results in uncontrolled (involuntary) movement of the head.

(4) *Vidhura Marma* — It is present below the lower part of pinna (Ear). These are two in number, present below both the ears. These are nerve-based *marmas*, measuring about 1/2 of the finger breadth and belongs to *vaikalyakara* group. Injury to this point causes deafness.

(5) *Phaṇa Marma* — These are present internally on either side of the nostrils, connecting with auditory canal (two in number). These are vessel-based *marmas*, measuring about 1/2 of the finger breadth and belongs to the *vaikalyakara* group. Injury to these points creates impairment (loss) of smell perception.

(6) *Apānga Marma* — These are present at the end of eyebrows below the outer angle of eyes on both sides (two in number). These are vessel-based *marmas*, measuring about 1/2 of the finger breadth and belong to *vaikalyakara* group. Injury to these points causes blindness.

(7) *Āvarta Marma* — These points are situated just above the tail end of eyebrows, particularly at the lower end of the forehead (two in

number). These are joint-based *marmas*, measuring about 1/2 of the fingers breadth and belong to *vaikalyakara* group. Injury to these points causes blindness or impairment of vision.

(8) *Sankha Marma* — These are present at the tail end of eyebrows in between the ears and forehead (two in number). These are bone-based *marmas*, measuring about 1/2 of the finger breadth and belong to *sadyaprāṇahara* group i.e. immediate death following injury or trauma.

(9) *Utkshepa Marma* — These are present above the *sankha marma* at the border of hairline (two in number). These are ligament-based marmas and belong to the *vishalyaghna* group that means the person can survive as long as the foreign body is remained embedded at the site. If the lodged foreign body will be extracted out, then the patient will die. The practitioner has to wait till the foreign body comes out after putrefaction.

(10) *Sthapanī Marma* — It is situated in between the two eyebrows and one in number. This is a vessel-based *marma*, measuring about 1/2 of the finger breadth and belongs to the *vishalyaghna* group, i.e. life continues till the lodged foreign body remains embedded at the site.

(11) *Simanta Marma* — These are five in number and situated inside the brain. These are joint-based *marmas*, which spread sideways and upwards and can be correlated with the brain sutures. They measure about four fingers each and belong to *kālāntara prāṇahara* group. Injury to these vital points causes insanity, giddiness, memory loss leading to death within one month.

(12) *Sringātaka Marma* — These are four in number and found at the junction of vessels supplying tongue, nose, eyes and ears above the palate. These are vessel-based *marmas*, measuring about four fingers each and belong to sadya *prāṇahara* group. Injury to these vital points causes sudden death.

(13) *Adhipati Marma* — This vital point is situated at above the meeting place of sinuses inside the brain, lining the inner side of the cranium. This is a joint-based *marma*, measuring about 1/2 of the finger breadth and belongs to sadya *parāṇahara* group. Injury to this vital point causes immediate death. This is one in number.

In this way, all the 37 vital points present in head and neck region are described.

2.6 Body Physiology in Ayurveda

The Ayurvedic concepts of physiology, pathology, diagnosis, prognosis and treatment, are all based upon the interplay of three humours (*tridosha* theory) in the body. The three humours (*tridosha*) are the biological form of five elements, which govern the physiological and pathological processes in the living body. They are not composed of all the five elements individually, rather collectively they form the five elements. Space and air are combined together to constitute the humour *vāta* whereas fire forms the humour *pitta*, and water and earth constitute the humour *kapha*, combinedly (Frawley and Lad, 1989).

Literally, the word *dosha* in Sanskrit means evening or darkness, otherwise "the blemish that transgresses". It signifies their ability to vitiate body tissues and organs to originate a bad consequence or detrimental effect to health. They are also called as *tridhātus* (three essential elements) as they support the body organs to maintain good health in their state of equilibrium. In another sense, the three humours have the ability to influence the functions of everything in human body, starting from a minute cell to tissues and glands. So, the treatment is nothing but to bring these three humours to a state of equilibrium and maintain this forever. Therefore, a harmonious state of three humours creates good health and disease occurs when this equilibrium is disturbed.

Literally, *Vāta* means movement and the power to carry things. It is a state of kinetic energy, that generates movement in body parts, organs, fluids, tissues and even cells. In a broader sense, it can be correlated with the activities of nervous system, both sympathetic and parasympathetic. Literally, the word *pitta* means temperature or heat energy. In living cells, it can be assumed to be the biological transformation of heat energy which includes activities of enzymes and hormones and the process of metabolism. Literally, the word *kapha* (*slesmā*) means binding ability or the process that holds things together. Thus, it can be correlated with the activities of tissue fluids and the process of anabolism. The humours *pitta* and *kapha* are potential in nature and get activated by the influence of humour *vāta* to perform their normal functions in body. It is just like the nerves, stimulating the glands and organs to secrete or release hormones, enzymes and other body fluids.

As described earlier, these three humours (*tridosha*) are the play masters of body physiology and pathology. In their subtle form, they are present in intracellular space and responsible for the secretion of neurohormones, which control all the life activities. In the gross form, *vata* is predominantly present in the space below umbilical region, *pitta* in between umbilical region and heart, and *kapha* in the space above the cardiac region. These are the principal sites for the three humours as they exist in each cell of the human body. The three humours exist in a cell in the aggregate and not as separate entities. The nucleus or central zone is the site of humour *kapha*, which is composed of earth and water in the five-element group. So, it is the heaviest part of a cell as earth and water are heavier than other elements. The middle zone or cytoplasm is the site of humour *pitta*, which is composed of the fire element. The fluidity of cytoplasm is due to the water element but the functions of cytoplasm are attributed to *pitta* due to its predominance. The outer zone or cell membrane is the site for the humour *vata*, which is composed of space and air elements. The porous structure of the cell membrane represents the elements space and air and lightest among cell structure as space and air are lightest among the five elements. The other suspended structures in cytoplasm like mitochondria, ribosome, golgi bodies, vacuole, etc. also represent the predominance of humours *viz.* mitochondria — *pitta*, vacuole — *vata* and ribosome — *kapha*, etc. It is a matter of great concern that the cell membrane plays an important role in activation of the cell including its functions. Alfred G. Gilman and Martin Rodbell were jointly awarded the Nobel Prize for Medicine in 1994 for their discovery of "G-proteins in cell membrane and their role in signal transduction in cells". G-proteins have been named so because they bind guanosine-5′-triphosphate (GTP). The two Nobel Laurates found the G-proteins to act as signal transducers like a switchboard, which transmit and modulate signals in cells. G-proteins have the ability to activate different cellular amplifier systems. They receive multiple signals from the exterior, integrate them and thus control fundamental life processes in the cells. This is the property attributed to the humour *vata*, which is activating and dynamic in nature. This is responsible for movement i.e. the activation of different cellular amplifier systems. Disturbances in the function of G-protein i.e. altered transduction of signals can lead to a diseased state. There are thousands of billions of cells in our body that act combinedly to allow us to perform our daily activities and to meet the challenges. This cooperation is achieved partly by cells communicating with each other through chemical signals. Earl Sutherland (USA) who had received the Nobel Prize in 1971, named these chemical signals that are used to communicate between the cells as "the first messenger". The first messenger is converted into a signal called "the second messenger" in the cell membrane. The second messenger acts inside the cell. The conversion of "first messenger" into "second messenger" involves a cooperative action of three different functional entities: *viz.* (1) a discriminator (receptor) that recognises different extracellular chemical signals (first messengers), (2) a transducer that provides a link between the discriminator and the amplifier and thus plays a key role in signal transduction, (need a GTP for action), (thus named as G-proteins) and (3) an amplifier that generates large quantities of second messenger intracellularly, for example, cyclic AMP. This is the discovery of Martin Rodbell for which he was awarded with the Nobel Prize. It may be assumed that the release of "the first messengers" is at level of *trigunas* or three energies (*sattva, raja* and *tama*) and the conversion and activation of "the second messengers" is at *tridosha* level or three humour level (*vāta, pitta* and *kapha*).

The functions of the discriminator (receptor) are somewhat similar to the functions of humour *kapha*, which is conserving in nature. Similarly, the functions of transducer can be compared with functions of *pitta*, which is transformative or supporting in nature. The functions of the amplifier can be compared with that of humour *vāta*, which is activating or creative in nature. This proves the interplay of three humours at every level starting from cellular to organic level.

The signal transducers usually require a GTP, an energy rich compound, for their action and thus, named as G-proteins. The nomenclature is given by Alfred G. Gilman. Interestingly, G-proteins are composed of three separate peptide chains of different length, each existing in multiple forms. They are denoted by alpha (α), beta (β) and gamma (γ), the first three letters of Greek alphabet. The alpha (α) subunit, which is the largest and most active can bind with GTP and activate the amplifiers to generate the second messengers that act inside the cell. This can be correlated with the functions of humour *vāta*, that activates the other two humours pitta and kapha for their corresponding functions. Without *vāta, they are inactive and their functions are controlled by the humour vāta.* These are all about the three humours in their subtle form at intracellular level. Now, we will discuss the functions of three humours in their gross form.

The three humours are responsible for all the life processes, both physiological and pathological. The interplay among themselves determines the state of health and disease. When one of the three humours increases, it tends other humours decrease simultaneously, resulting a pathological condition. At different stages, there is predominance of one of the three humours, that may or may not affect the functions of other humours.

2.7 Predominance of Humours at Different Stages

Stage	*Kapha*	*Pitta*	*Vāta*
Age	Childhood and young age (up to 25 years)	Middle age (25–60 years)	Old age (above 60 years)
Daytime	Morning	Noon	Afternoon
Night	Evening	Mid-night	Before sunrise
Digestion	After ingestion of food but before the process of digestion	During the process of digestion	After the process of digestion

Naturally, the three humours get accumulated, vitiated and pacified at different seasons in a year. The accumulation occurs at their principal sites, and this is the start of pathogenesis. Diseases with prominent signs and symptoms appear at the time of vitiation. Then, the vitiated humours get pacified naturally (if the amount of vitiation is less) or need treatment (if the amount of vitiation is more), which is done at the time of vitiation of humours.

Humours	Time of accumulation	Time of vitiation	Time of pacification
Vāta	Summer	Rainy	Autumn
Pitta	Rainy	Autumn	Winter
Kapha	Early winter	Spring	Summer

Vāta — *Vāta* comprises the activities of nervous system. It is the prime moving force in our body and is responsible for the processes of respiration, circulation, digestion, transportation of nutrients and elimination of waste products. It is the most powerful and influential humour because it acts as the driving force for the other two humours, seven structural body tissues, waste products and also responsible for movement of body parts and function of organs. In the most ancient treatise of Ayurveda, i.e. *Charak Samhita*, *Vāta* is described as *Tantrayantradhara* that means it holds up (responsible) all the systems and organs of the body. Other functions of the humour *vāta* are (as described in *Charak Samhita*):

(1) It provides the initiation to the upward, downward, inward and outward movements.
(2) Activates and controls the functions of mind.
(3) Employs all the sense organs in their activities. (five sense organs in Ayurveda *viz.* organs of vision — eyes, organs of smell — nose, organs of hearing — ears, organ of tastes perception — tongue, and organ of tactile stimulation — skin).
(4) Carries all the sense perceptions — sound, touch, sight, taste and smell.
(5) Causes structural formation of all the body tissues (*dhātu*) and organs.
(6) Promotes the union of body and holds together different parts.
(7) Initiates the speech.
(8) Originates sound and touch perception (as *vāta* is composed of space and air elements; sound and touch are the subtle elements of space and air).
(9) Root of the auditory and tactile sensation.
(10) Source of exhilaration and courage.
(11) Stimulates the digestive fire and regulates digestion.
(12) Absorbs the vitiated humours.
(13) Expels the waste products out of the body.
(14) Creates the gross and minute channels of the body.
(15) Mould the shape of the embryo.
(16) Determines the life span.

These are the functions of humour *vāta* in its unvitiated state. When is gets vitiated, all its functions become disturbed, causing illness. There are five divisions of the humour *vāta viz. prāṇa, udāna, vyāna, samāna* and *apāna*. The five-fold division if based upon the site, movement, direction and functions of the humour *vāta*.

A. *Prāṇa vāta* — Literally, *prāṇa* means "forward moving air". The prime abode of *prāṇa vāyu* is head and chest, and it moves through throat, tongue, mouth and nose. It is mainly concerned with respiration, both inhalation and exhalation. Its associated functions are ingestion of food and water, act of spitting, sneezing and belching. *Prāṇa vāta* is the form of physical and mental energy, that gives vitality to the physical body and provides power to think.

B. *Udānā vāta* — Literally, *udānā* means "upwards moving air". Its main site is head and thorax (*uras*). Its primary functions are initiation of speech, motivation for work, and conservation of life energy. It is the positive energy that provides us the enthusiasm and will to speak, think and perform. It also controls the functions of five senses *viz.* eyes, ears, tongue, nose and skin. When *Udānā vāta* gets vitiated, the patient finds it difficult to co-ordinate, balance and integrate the sensory and motor nerves. It is also associated with memory and intellect.

C. *Vyāna vāta* — Literally, vyāna means "outward moving air" that means it moves from the centre to periphery. It pervades all over the body though its primary site is heart. It is primarily concerned about the circulation of blood (*rasa* and *rakta dhātu*) at all levels. It initiates the heart to pump (beat) the blood and provides energy for it. It is responsible for five kinds of action i.e. contraction, expansion, upward movement, downward movement, and walking or other general movements. It also controls blinking of eyes, yawning, and sweating (perspiration). Since, It is present all over the body, it assists other varieties of *vāta* in their work and acts as a reserve source of energy for them.

D. *Samāna vāta* — Literally, *samāna* means "equal" that means "the balancing air". It is situated in abdomen, primarily at naval region. *Samāna vāta* is responsible for the process of digestion and metabolism. It coordinates and motivates the organs of digestion such as stomach, pancreas, liver and small intestine in their work for an effective digestion. It also separates the pure nutrients from the waste products of digestion and later forms the urine, stool and sweat. It also helps in the formation of seven structural elements (*sapta dhātu*).

E. *Apāna vāta* — Literally, *apāna* means "air that moves away". Its primary site is the pelvic region or the region below naval. It is responsible for the elimination of urine, faeces, gas, menstrual blood, etc. Its function also includes production of semen and ovum, performance of sexual act, movement of spermatozoa into the uterus, fertilisation, holding the foetus inside the uterus until delivery and expulsion of foetus during delivery. This means, that the whole process of procreation is controlled and regulated by this *apāna vāta.* Vitiation of this *vāta* creates a number of diseases, which include diseases of urinary tract, kidney, renal calculi, constipation, diarrhoea, piles, fistula, infertility, impotence, production of vitiated semen, menstrual disorders, lack of interest in sexual act and genetic disorders, etc.

In short, the function of all the five divisions of *vāta* can be summarised in a cyclic order. *Prāna vāta* governs the intake of food along with respiration. *Samāna vāta* is responsible for the digestion. *Vyāna vāta* governs the circulation of nutrients and *udāna vāta* is responsible for the release of positive energy from it. And lastly, *apāna vāta* governs the elimination of waste products of digestion. All the five divisions are interlinked and perform combinedly for the maintenance of good health. When anyone of these *vātas* gets disturbed, it compel others to be disturbed and thus, creates the disease. Of these divisions, *Prāna vāta* is most important and it provides strength to other divisions to perform their functions.

2.8 Vitiation of *Vāta Dosha* and Treatment

Generally, *vāta* gets vitiated by two ways *viz.* (1) loss of structural elements (*dhātus*) and (2) obstruction in the transporting channels, impeding the free flow of *vāta* inside it. Again, the loss of structural elements or *dhātus* is of two types — i.e. (a) *Anuloma kşaya* — Successive loss in the ascending order i.e. from *rasa dhātu* to *sukra dhātu* (blood plasma to reproductive tissue). This is resulted from less intake of nutritious food, altered digestion, defects in absorption and due to disorders of gastro intestinal tract. (b) *Pratiloma kşaya* — Reverse loss of structural elements in the descending order i.e. from *sukra dhātu* to *rasa dhātu* (from reproductive tissue to blood plasma). This occurs due to excessive sexual act, losing maximum amount of semen.

The humour *vāta* is increased due to excessive intake of dry, cold, light foods, foods with the taste of pungent, bitter and astringent and excess physical exercise and physical work. It is decreased due to more intake of sweet, sour foods, heavy and oily foods and less physical exercise. Signs and symptoms of increased *vāta* are emaciation, blackish discolouration of skin, tremor, loss of consciousness, insomnia, loss of body strength, impairment of sense organs, pain in bones, parching of bone marrow and synovial fluid, constipation, flatulence, delusion, timidity, fear, grief, delirium, etc. Signs and symptoms of decreased *vāta* are excessive salivation, anorexia, nausea, loss of consciousness, delusion, low speech, decreased physical activity, sorrow, loss of appetite, disorders of digestive fire, etc. Signs and symptoms of vitiated *vāta* are unwanted movement, tremor, restricted movement, body ache, pain in bone and joints, impairment of sense organs, hyperactivity, loss of concentration, delirium, different types of cutting, splitting, poking, squeezing, tearing, gnawing, spasmodic pain all over the body, fear, anxiety, feeling of insecure, loss of libido, insomnia, bitter taste in mouth, hoarseness of voice, tinnitus, excessive yawning, abdominal distention, etc.

Therapeutic enema and medicated oils are considered best treatment for the disorder of *vāta*. Food and medicine of sweet, sour and salt taste, drugs of hot potency and unctuousness are also used for alleviation of *vāta* disorders. Oleation and hot fomentation with *vāta* pacifying herbs are advised for relief of pain.

Pitta — The humour *pitta* is composed of fire element and balancing or transformative in nature. It generates the heat energy and helps in metabolism. The functions of *pitta* can be correlated with that of hormones and enzymes of our body. The functions of *pitta*, in its unvitiated state, are:

(1) The complete process of metabolism i.e. digestion, absorption, assimilation, etc.
(2) Production and maintenance of body temperature.
(3) Production of hunger and thirst.
(4) Responsible for vision.
(5) Regulates the colour, complexion and lustre of body (skin, eyes).
(6) Intelligence.
(7) Power of comprehension.
(8) Valour or bravery.
(9) Ambition or desire to prosper in life.
(10) Softness of the body parts.

(11) Natural tendency of hate, anger, jealously.
(12) Cheerfulness and lucidity of mind.

Primarily, *pitta* resides in stomach, small intestine, liver, pancreas, sweat glands, blood, fat, eyes and skin. Its chief site is the region in between heart and umbilicus. There are also five divisions of *pitta viz. pāchaka, ranjaka, sādhaka, alochaka, bhrājaka.*

(1) *Pāchaka pitta* — Literally, it means "that digests". It is responsible for digestion and metabolism. It is situated in stomach, small intestine and pancreas. After digestion, it separates pure nutrient fluid from the waste products. It is the chief among all the five divisions of *pitta* and provides strength to other *pittas* for their normal function.
(2) *Ranjaka pitta* — Literally, *Ranjaka* means "to put colours". Its principal site is liver. It gives the characteristic red colour to the blood, i.e. formation of *rakta dhātu* from *rasa dhātu*. This function can be correlated with haemopoiesis.
(3) *Sādhaka pitta* — Literally, *Sadhaka* means "effective of or promoting". It is situated in the heart (*hridaya*) and associated with the mental attributes like memory, intelligence, comprehension, self-confidence, etc. All these mental activities are directly correlated to the cerebral cortex, thalamus and hypothalamus. But, Ayurveda considers heart to be the site of mind and that is why, ascribed all these functions to *sādhaka pitta* present in heart. It is very difficult to identify any substance or substances, which have all the functions that are ascribed to *sādhaka pitta* in Ayurveda. For a correlation, it could be acetylcholine, on which movement of nerve impulses depends.
(4) *Alochaka pitta* — Literally, *Alochaka* means "that supports vision". Its principal site is in eyes and is responsible for vision. The chemical changes, that take place when light falls on retina (rhodopsin to scotopsin, retinal, etc.) and transmission of nerve impulses to the visual area of cerebral cortex (occipital lobe — brodmann area 17) may be attributed to *alochaka pitta*. Furthermore, it is divided into two types *viz.* (i) *Chakşu vaiseshika* and (ii) *Buddhi vaiseshika. Chakşu vaiseshika alochaka pitta* is concerned with vision. *Buddhi vaiseshika alochaka pitta* is responsible for the knowledge, power of reasoning, logical skill,

etc. It can be correlated with the hormone melatonin, secreted by the pineal gland. Both these two types of *alochaka pitta* are inter-related, which is evident and proved from the fact that synthesis and secretion of melatonin are dramatically affected by light exposure to the eyes. The hormone melatonin has the light transducing ability to communicate with cells, tissues and organs of human body and thus, controls the circadian rhythms (biological clock). Serum concentration of melatonin is low during day time and increases to a peak in night and darkness. In other mammals, it also controls the reproductive function. But, the functions of *Buddhi vaiseshika alochaka pitta* (melatonin) and the pineal gland (*Ājnā chakra*) in Ayurveda means a lot more. In Ayurveda, pineal gland is named as *Ājnā chakra* and regarded as the site of mind. Even French philosopher. *Rene Descartes* (1596–1650) admitted it as "the seat of the soul". It is believed in Ayurveda that one would be able to develop telepathic communication by activating *Ājnā chakra* through meditation. One recent study showed definite surge in melatonin hormone after a period of successful meditation. Nobel laureate Julius Axelrod (1970) has already described melatonin as a chemically converted form of the active neurotransmitter serotonin, which is stored along with norepinephrine in nerve terminals for later release. He discovered the functions of melatonin as a powerful neurotransmitter, when released through the central nervous system. A recent study by Dr. David Klein, chief Neuroendocrinology, National Institute of Child Health and Human Development (NICHD) USA suggests detoxifying activities of melatonin in the retina, which may further increase the understanding of eye diseases and sleep disorders. More studies should be done in this regard to understand the function of melatonin in alleviating mental stress, improving immunity, preventing cancer, Alzheimer's disease, Parkinson's disease and senile dementia and regulating the biological clock.

(5) *Bhrājaka pitta* — *Bhrājaka pitta* is situated in the skin. It is responsible for normal skin pigmentation, lustre and maintenance of body temperature. Insulation and temperature regulation property of skin is attributed to *bhrājaka pitta.* It's another function is skin lustre and normal skin pigmentation, which is believed to be the function of melanin, secreted by the melanocyte cells present in the skin. In this

connection, diseases like melanoma, albinism, leukoderma, hyperpigmentation, basal cell carcinoma, etc. can be treated by pacifying *bhrājaka pitta* in Ayurvedic parlance.

2.9 Vitiation of *Pitta Dosha* and Treatment

Pitta dosha is generally increased and got vitiated by taking excess pungent, sour and salty foods, excessive exposure to sun and heat, excess mental stress and strain, anger, frustration, faulty dietary habits like overeating, untimely eating, eating before the digestion of previous meal, fasting, excess intake of certain items like sesamum oil, mustard oil, curd, cow gram, *Linum usitatissimum*, unnatural mode of sexual indulgence, awakening at night, etc.

Increased *pitta* causes yellowish discolouration of skin and eyes, fatigue, feeling of discomfort, weakness in sense organs, burning sensation in stomach, hunger, thirst, sleeping disorders, anger, excessive sweating and sour taste in mouth. The humours are increased at their principal sites and then got vitiated by being excited by certain causes. Vitiated humours spread out to different body parts and cause diseases. Vitiated humour *pitta* causes fever, diarrhoea, heart burn, burning sensation in stomach, mouth, throat, increased thirst, hunger, hyperacidity, blood disorders, skin diseases, ulcerations, excess foul discharge from external openings, blurred vision, boils, anger, impatience, discontent, irritability, sleep disorders, mental confusion, etc. Decreased *Pitta* may cause indigestion, anorexia, body stiffness, coldness, irregular pains, tremors, and whitish discolouration of skin, nails, eyes, etc.

Therapeutic purgation and medicated cow's ghee are considered best treatment in *pitta* aggravation. Intake of food and medicines of sweet, bitter and astringent taste is considered as a good remedy for *pitta dosha.* Herbal medicines processed with cow's milk and cow's ghee are also administered. Slightly warm food with moderately heavy foods should be consumed and pungent sour, salty foods, pickles, should be avoided.

Kapha — The humour *kapha* is composed of water and earth in the five-element group and conserving or stabilising (*tāmasika*) in nature. It provides the structural integrity and is responsible for coordination of body systems. Functions of *kapha* can be correlated with the functions of tissue fluids, anabolism and skeletal system. Primarily, *kapha* resides in chest, head, neck, throat, joints, stomach, tongue, nose and adipose tissue (fat). However, its chief site is the chest region. Functions of *kapha*, in its unvitiated state, can be summarised as below:

(1) Provides stability to body.
(2) Promotes unctuousness or lubrication (soothing effect).
(3) Responsible for compactness and well functioning of joints.
(4) Regulates the immune system and provides natural tissue resistance.
(5) Responsible for virility (sexual potency) and reproduction.
(6) Tissue building and wound healing (repair process).
(7) Supports memory retention (*dhruti*).
(8) Gives the biological strength and vigour.
(9) Cause of heaviness and courage.
(10) Forgiveness or forbearance.
(11) Absence of greediness.
(12) More emotional attachment and calmness.

Again, the humour *kapha* is divided into five sub-types, each of which has separate functions. They are — *avalambaka kapha, kledaka kapha, tarpaka kapha, bodhaka kapha* and *sleshmaka kapha.* Their site and important functions are described below.

A. *Avalambaka kapha* — Literally, it means the agent "that protects, guards, defends or governs". It is present in the chest region and considered as the body's store house of *kapha.* It provides strength to other divisions of *kapha* for their proper functioning. This *kapha* protects and governs the functions of heart and lungs (*trika* — three structures). It promotes and facilitates proper functioning of heart and lungs. It can be compared with the interstitial fluid in the extra cellular space.
B. *Kledaka kapha* — Literally, *kledaka* means "that moistens". Its principal site is stomach (*Āmāśaya*). It is responsible for moistening, disintegration and break down of food particles in the stomach. It can be correlated with the mucous secretions of stomach, which helps in digestion.
C. *Tarpaka kapha* — Literally, *tarpaka* means "that nourishes". It is located in the head (brain). It nourishes the brain and enables it to perform effectively. It also nourishes the centres of sense organs in brain and

facilitates their action. It can be correlated with the cerebrospinal fluid (CSF), which has almost the same function.

D. *Bodhaka kapha* — Literally, *bodhaka* means "that provides knowledge or perception, communicates or reminds". It is present in the tongue and responsible for taste perception. It also lubricates the food and make it suitable for easy deglutition. It also moist the vocal cords and enables sound production. It can be compared with the saliva secretions of mouth.
E. *Sleshaka kapha* — Literally, *sleshaka* means "that binds or lubricates". It is present in all joints of our body. It is responsible for the integrity of the joints and their proper functioning. It provides lubrication to the joints. *Sleshaka kapha* remains inside the *sleshmadharā kalā*, which covers all bone joints. Thus, it can be compared with the synovial fluid, which is responsible for joint lubrication. It also acts as a cementing substance and protects the joints from friction, trauma and injury.

2.10 Vitiation of *Kapha Dosha* and Treatment

The humour *kapha* is generally increased and gets vitiated by taking food predominant of sweet, sour and salty taste, taking more heavy, oily, cold, slimy, unctuous food, excess intake of milk and milk products, excess intake of meat and sea foods, intake of sweets produced from cane-sugar, adopting sedentary life style, excess sleep, lack of exercise, sleeping after taking lunch, overeating and eating before the digestion of previous meal.

Increased *kapha* causes coldness, weight gain, oedema, whitish discolouration, laziness, heaviness, debility of body parts, obstruction of transporting channels, fainting, drowsiness, excess sleep, asthmatic attack (difficulty in breathing), cough, excess salivation, nausea, loss of appetite, looseness of joints, etc. Increased *kapha* gets vitiated, when it comes across synergistic climatic factors and other favourable conditions. Vitiated (aggravated) *kapha* causes weight gain, obesity, diabetes, asthma, cough, nausea, fever, oedema, excess salivation and congestion in chest and throat, pale, cold skin, weakness of joints, oedema, depressed mental attitude, lethargic, apathetic dull thinking, sweet taste in mouth, etc. Decreased *Kapha* may cause giddiness, confusion, bodyache, insomnia, burning sensation, pricking pain, feeling of burning, bursting, churning and movement of hot fumes inside, looseness of joints, palpitation, emptiness at the sites of *kapha*, etc.

Therapeutic vomiting and honey are considered best treatments in vitiation of *kapha dosha*. Food and medicine, predominance of pungent, bitter and astringent taste are also administered. Warm, light food devoid of butter and more spicy should be given. Milk and dairy products, meat, sea foods, oils, sugars are to be avoided. Mild to moderate exercise, mild exposure to sun and sweating (sudation) using *kapha* pacifying herbs are beneficial. Herbs that pacify *kapha* are *piper nigrum*, *piper lonum*, *zingiber officinale*, *plumbago zeylanica*, *cordial dichotoma*, *curcuma longa*, *onosma bracteatum*, *Dhatura metel*, *solanum surattense*, *myrica esculenta*, etc.

Similar to the humours, the sub-humours (sub-*doshas*) also work together and form organic systems combinedly. *Prāṇa vata*, *sādhaka pitta* and *avalambaka kapha* are related to heart and lungs and responsible for proper functioning of respiratory and cardiovascular systems. They also regulate mental functions. *Udāna vāta*, *alochaka pitta* and *tarpaka kapha* are related to brain, spinal cord, nervous system and sense organs. They are also responsible for intelligence, memory, speech and vision. *Samāna vāta*, *pāchaka pitta* and *kledaka kapha* are related to the digestive system. They regulate the processes of digestion, absorption, assimilation and formation of elementary tissues from purest form of digestion. *Vyāna vāta*, *ranjaka pitta* and *bodhaka kapha* help in digestion, but particularly related to the formation of blood and its circulation to each part of body. *Apāna vāta*, *bhrājaka pitta* and *sleshaka kapha* are related to the excretion, skin lustre and wellness of joints and extremities.

2.11 Some Reflections

Ancient medicine never has detailed anatomical or structural descriptions about the body structures. Unlike modern medicine which builds up and establishes its management policy according to structural details of the tissues and organs concerned, together with their apparent functional derangements, ancient medicine like Ayurveda and Chinese medicine rely on philosophical basis and general observations. Structural considerations might more frequently follow, rather than precede decision making. The structural descriptions of body organs and tissues in Ayurveda have indications that the information is based on surface knowledge of the human body. Such information is relevant to management plan which, however, is mainly governed by relevant traditional beliefs pertaining to the symptoms manifested. Structural considerations follows general planning.

The Ayurveda concept of conduit systems which are channels within the organs and tissues as well as interlinking facilities somewhat resembles the TCM concept of "meridians". A simplified version of the complicated network is convenient for management planning. The *marma* sites might resemble the acupoints along the meridian which, however, are never considered as vulnerable.

As long as the ancient teachings are not rigidly observed today, they could contribute greatly in modern medical practice.

References

Acharya, Y.T. (2001). *Ayurved Dipika Commentary of Chakrapani on Charak Samhita*, 5th Edition. Choukhambha Sanskrit Sansthan, Varanasi, India.

Chattopadhyaya, D. (1977). *Science and Society in Ancient India.* B.R. Grüner Publishing Company, Netherlands.

Dharmalingam, V., Radhika, M., Balasubramanian, A.V. (1991). *Marma Chikitsa in Traditional Medicine.* Lok Swaasthya Parampara Samvardhan Samithi, Madras.

Frawley, D. and Lad, V. (1989). *The Yoga of Herbs: An Ayurvedic Guide to Herbal Medicine.* Lotus Press, USA.

Shastri, A. (1997). *Ayurved Tatwa Sandipika commentary on Sushrut Samhita*, 11th Edition. Choukhambha Sanskrit Sansthan, Varanasi, India.

Tripathy, B. (1998). *Charak Chandrika Commentary on Charak Samhita*, 5th Edition. Chowkhamba Surbharti Prakashan, Varanasi, India.

Tripathy, B. (2003). *Nirmala Hindi Commentary on Astanga Hridaya*, 1st Edition Chowkhambha Sanskrit Pratisthan, Delhi, India.

Chapter 3

Health and Disease in Ayurveda

Debashis Panda

Abstract

Ayurveda and Chinese medicine has quite similar concept of health and disease. Each person has a separate body constitution in physical, mental, emotional and spiritual faculties. So, the treatment is individual specific and not common as in the case of modern medicine. Ayurveda and Traditional Chinese Medicine (TCM) practitioners treats the patient, not the disease and thus, assures a complete cure. Equilibrium in three humours, seven structural elements and proper evacuation of three waste products ensures good health and imbalance causes disease. The traditional medical practitioner has to maintain the equilibrium for a good health.

Keywords: Health; Disease; Environment; Balance; Pathogenesis; Homeostasis.

3.1 Introduction

The ancient oriental systems of medicine, Ayurveda and Chinese medicine, have quite similar concepts of health and disease. Each human being is considered as a miniature replica of the universe (macrocosm) in both systems of medicine. They believe in individuality i.e. each person has a separate body constitution in physical, mental, emotional and spiritual faculties. Each human being (microcosm) is characterised by a constant and dynamic interaction between the internal body organs with the environment or universe (macrocosm). As long as there is balance, good health continues. The disturbances in this homeostasis form the basis of pathogenesis. Health is the order and disease is the disorder. Irrespective of modern Western medicine, each disease is presented differently in different individuals and requires a unique mode of approach for each individual. For example, in Western medicine, "fever" is common to each patient and antipyretic agents act as universal antipyretic media in all cases. In contrast, "fever" is considered different among different patients in the oriental system of medicine and needs different medication for treatment in each case. In general, Western medicine treats the disease, whereas oriental medicine treats the sick.

The oriental systems of medicine, Ayurveda and Chinese medicine, do not consider body, mind and soul as separate entities, but as a whole continuum. It has been observed that mental and emotional states have significant influences on the physical health and *vice versa*. So, optimum health is considered as a state of physical, mental and spiritual well-being, not merely the physical health. This definition of health is not different from what the World Health Organization (WHO) advocates today. More descriptively, the definition of health, as cited by the ancient Indian sages, encompasses the following details:

(1) All the three humours must be in equilibrium.
(2) The digestive fire (*agni*) must be normal, leading to proper digestion, absorption and assimilation (physical health).
(3) The seven structural components (tissues — *dhātus*) must be in normal state and in integration with each other (physical health).
(4) Proper elimination of the waste products (physical health).
(5) The person must feel contented and exhilarated (spiritual health).
(6) Both sensory and motor organs must function normally and be coordinated properly (social health).
(7) There must be happiness in mind. The mental activities must be providing peace and calmness (mental health).

It is obvious that not only physical health, but spiritual, social and mental health are emphasised. The three humours act at all levels and control the overall functions. The coordinated equilibrium of the three humours is a sign of good health. Disturbances in any of the criteria listed above initiate imbalance in the equilibrium of the three humours, which later lead to the pathogenesis of a disease.

3.2 *Ayurvedic View of Diseases*

Diseases in Ayurveda are classified into seven broad categories and each category is further subdivided into two sub-groups basing upon the aetiological factors. Depiction of different types of diseases is as follows:

3.2.1 *Genetic (Ādibalapravritta)*

In Ayurvedic view, genetic disorders arise due to defects or impurities in the sperm or ovum of parents. The impurities may cause genetic diseases like diabetes, asthma, haemorrhoids, tuberculosis, skin diseases, etc. These are of two types; one arising from impurities found in the sperm of father (*Pitrija*) and another arising from impurities found in the ovum of mother (*Mātrija*). Impurities in sperm or ovum exist because of generally misconduct, defective dietary regimens, addiction, mental imbalance and stressful living. These disorders can be prevented by purifying the sperm and ovum of parents before conception.

3.2.2 *Congenital (Janmabalapravritta)*

These diseases are due to nutritional deficiencies in pregnancy (*rasakrita*) and unfulfilled desires of the expected mother during pregnancy (*dauhrida vimānaja*). *Janmabalapravritta* diseases include kyphosis, dwarfism, blindness, albinism, leukoderma, gigantism and other congenital anomalies. Even now-a-days, it is considered that congenital anomalies occur because of bad conduct practised by the pregnant mother and/or unfavourable food or drugs taken by the pregnant mother.

3.2.3 *Constitutional (Doshabalapravritta)*

The constitutional diseases arise due to the dietary and behavioural incompatibilities practised by the individuals. These cause imbalance in the coordinated equilibrium of the three humours, which leads to the diseased state. The constitutional diseases are of two types: somatic (*sāririka*) and psychic (*mānasika*).

Furthermore, the diseases could be *vātik*, *paittik*, or *sleshmik* in the somatic category and *rājasika* or *tāmasika* in the *psychic* category.

3.2.4 *Traumatic* (*Sanghātabalapravritta*)

Traumatic diseases occur due to the trauma produced by external or internal causes. These disorders are of two types i.e. external (*āgantuja*) or internal (*nija*) depending upon the nature of trauma. External trauma is induced by sharp or blunt instruments, fall, bites of animals or venomous insects. Internal trauma is caused by grief, fear, anger, jealousness or over stresses and strains. In both cases, imbalance in the equilibrium of the three humours is essential to bring about the diseased state. For internal trauma, loss of equilibrium occurs first, followed by the manifestations of the disease. In contrast, imbalance of the three humours is secondary to the occurrence of external injuries.

3.2.5 *Seasonal* (*Kālabalapravritta*)

These are diseases developed during changes in seasons and abnormal climatic conditions. These are also of two types; one group of diseases occurs at the climax of seasonal changes and another group of diseases occur during abnormal climatic conditions i.e. cold in summer or hot in winter. Ayurveda has advised special attention to be taken in the transitional period (*ritusandhi*) that occurs between two seasons. *Ritusandhi* (transitional period) is a period of 14 days comprising the last week of the outgoing season and the first week of the upcoming season. The seasonal change is usually gradual. Diseases like fever, influenza, headache, malaise, and cough occur in this period while already existing diseases get aggravated. Therefore, special care should be taken to avoid seasonal ailments. During this transitional period, the dietary and behavioural regimen for the outgoing season should be tapered off gradually while the regimen for the upcoming season is gradually introduced.

3.2.6 *Infections and Natural Calamities* (*Daivajanya*)

Daivajanya diseases are also of two types. One group of diseases is caused by infection of invading pathogens, bacteria, virus, fungus and parasites. Although these pathogens (bacteria, virus, etc.) were not known to the ancient sages of Ayurveda, they considered that these diseases were the result of some supernatural forces. They thought these diseases could be the results of sins and bad things done by the person involving current or previous lives. Another group of diseases is caused by natural calamities like earthquake, tsunami, flood, etc. Epidemic diseases are also included.

3.2.7 *Natural diseases* (*svabhāvabalapravritta*)

There are some diseases, which are inevitable and are sure to occur in every person apparently healthy. Ayurveda names them as natural diseases and these are hunger, thirst, sleep, senility and death.

3.3 Causes of Diseases in Ayurveda

Before starting the treatment, it is essential to find out the root cause of the disease. Unlike Western medicine, Ayurveda treats the root cause of the disease. Understanding the cause of a disease in Ayurveda is profound, yet simple. Ayurveda emphasises on three primary causes of diseases, i.e. inappropriate association of sense organs (*asātmyendriyārtha samyoga*), improper use of intellect and cognitive faculties (*Prajnāparādha*) and vagaries of time or distorted rhythms of nature (*kāla parināma*). The balanced state of these three factors i.e. proper involvement of sense organs, intellect and natural rhythms of nature is a sign of good health. In contrast, excessive, inadequate and improper transgression of these factors are capable of vitiating the three humours and thus, serves as the root cause of all diseases.

3.3.1 *Asātmyendriyārthā Samyoga* (*Improper or Unaccustomed Contact of Sense Organs*)

There are 10 sense organs in Ayurveda, out of which five are sensory sense organs and another five are motor sense organs. Five sensory sense organs are ears, skin, eyes, tongue and nose; meanwhile, motor sense organs are hands, legs, organ of speech, organ of excretion (anus) and organ of procreation. All the organs are activated for perception or action by the presence of mind in them. Therefore, an unwholesome perception or action produces an unwholesome effect in the mind, which is vulnerable for the pathogenesis of a certain disease. The improper or unwholesome contact can be of three types *viz.* excessive, inadequate or distorted. For example, seeing very bright light or contemplating objects for a longer period is considered as excessive contact of the sense of vision (eye). Seeing an object in excessive dim light or darkness or not seeing any object is considered as inadequate contact of the sense of vision (eye). Seeing objects which are frightening, fearful, strange, shocking or abnormal is considered as distorted or improper contact of the sense of vision.

The excessive, inadequate or distorted contacts of other sense organs are similarly assessed.

3.3.2 *Prajnāparādha (Improper Use of Intellect or Cognitive Faculties)*

Intellect is a combined process of three cognitive faculties, *viz.* power of acquisition (*dhi*), power of retention (*dhruti* — keeping something in memory) and power of re-collection (*smruti*). When these three cognitive attitudes of a person are destroyed or superimposed by ignorance and negligence, a false awareness is created, which impels the person to evil thoughts and deeds. Thus, *prajnāparādha* can be translated as "false awareness" or "volitional transgression". This causes vitiation of all the three humours and forms the basis of all diseases.

Prajnāparādha is of three types *viz.* physical, speech and mental, which again can be sub-divided into excessive, inadequate and distorted types. Different activities of each category are depicted in the following table:

Prajnāparādha	Sub-types	Activities
(1) Physical (*kāyika*)	Excessive	Excessive work, exercise or sexual activity.
	Inadequate	Less or no physical activity.
	Distorted	Suppression or initiation of natural urges, improper posture, endangered activities.
(2) Speech (*vācika*)	Excessive	Talking or speaking Loud or for long periods.
	Inadequate	Talking little or maintaining silence for long periods.

(*Continued*)

(*Continued*)

Prajnāparādha	Sub-types	Activities
	Distorted	Telling lies, untrue, irrelevant, or using impolite, abusive and quarrelsome words.
(3) Mental (*mānasika*)	Excessive	Excessive thinking or continuing mental activities for long periods.
	Inadequate	Making little or no use of mental faculties.
	Distorted	Anxiety, tension, fear, grief, anger, greed, lust, jealousness.

3.3.3 *Parināma* (*Vagaries of Time and Weather*)

The body has to make adjustment with the changing climatic and weather conditions. When this adjustment fails or if there are unexpected vagaries of time, homeostasis gets disturbed and gives rise to pathogenesis of a disease. There are again three types, *viz.* excessive, inadequate and distorted. Excessive type corresponds to oppressive climatic conditions which are far away from normal, e.g. extreme heat in summer causing sun stroke and freezing cold in winter causing frost bite.

Inadequate type refers to the diminished features of a season like less rain in rainy season or less cold in winter season. Distorted weather corresponds to different seasonal conditions or abnormal features, e.g. cold in summer and hot in winter. In addition, different stages of life (childhood, middle age, old age, etc.) have different needs and require unique care and attention. Any imbalance to these requirements may cause disturbance in the three humours which later form the base of a disease.

In simple words, all the diseases originate in the mind first, and then affect the three humours. Later, the affected three humours vitiate the body tissues and organs resulting in diseases.

Followers of Ayurveda advocate the following causes as the common aetiology of all diseases.

(1) **Unwholesome food and irregular eating habits:** Unwholesome food refers to those not suitable or favourable to the body and mind.

Irregular eating habits include taking food either before or after scheduled time and taking excessive or insufficient food.

(2) **Suppression of natural urges:** Human body is a biological machine that requires continuous supply of air, food and water for existence and proper functioning. The metabolic wastes produced as the result should be excreted in time to avoid toxic retention. Every individual has to take sufficient rest and sleep at regular intervals to replenish the loss incurred during life activities. These types of biological needs are called as natural urges, essential for the maintenance of life processes and should not be suppressed by any means. These are:

(i) Passage of gas through anus (flatus).
(ii) Passage of stool (defecation).
(iii) Passage of urine (micturition).
(iv) Sneezing.
(v) Thirst.
(vi) Hunger.
(vii) Sleep (biological rest at night).
(viii) Coughing.
(ix) Exertional breathlessness.
(x) Yawning.
(xi) Tears (following sorrow or happiness).
(xii) Vomiting.
(xiii) Semen (ejaculation).

All the above urges are natural and are controlled by the most powerful humour *vāta* i.e. the nervous system. Voluntary suppression of these natural urges causes obstruction in the free flow of the humour *vāta* and thus, aggravates it. Later, the aggravated *vāta* causes vitiation of the other two humours i.e. *pitta* and *kapha* and gives rise to diseases. At the same time, artificial induction of these urges is equally harmful and forms the base in the pathogenesis of other diseases.

However, there are certain mental urges which should be suppressed for the betterment of health. These are anger, greed, jealousy, hatred, lust, fear, etc. One should always suppress these impulses or emotions to cool down the mind and enjoy a peaceful healthy life.

(3) **Awakening at night and day sleep:** Awakening at night and day sleep are other causes that form the basis of pathogenesis. An individual should go to sleep before 9 p.m. and get up before 5 a.m. in the morning. Thus, the saying, "Early to bed and early to rise, makes a man healthy, wealthy and wise." Remaining awakened at night aggravates the *vāta* and *pitta* humours whereas taking day sleep aggravates all the three humours *vāta, pitta* and *kapha.*

(4) **Excessive sexual indulgence:** It is another cause responsible for the pathogenesis. The excessive loss of semen in sexual act causes loss of the preceding *dhātus* (structural elements) in the descending order starting from the semen (*sukra dhātu*) to lymphatic tissue (*rasa dhātu*). Loss of the structural tissues vitiates the *vāta* humour and later the vitiated *vāta* aggravates the other two humours, *pitta* and *kapha,* and form the basis of pathogenesis. For this reason, Ayurveda experts advocate the saving of semen in order to lead a healthy and long life. They recommend sexual emission once in three days in all seasons except summer season, where it should be once in 15 days (fortnightly). Ayurveda believes that neuromuscular disorders, pain, cough, asthma, fever, general debility, anaemia, tuberculosis, epilepsy and other neurological diseases may occur due to excessive indulgence in sexual acts. Therefore, one should save semen (*sukra dhātu*) to lead a healthy and long life. By practising abstinence, one can get longevity, delayed aging, strength, lustre, good health and well developed body muscles.

3.4 Concept of *Agni* and Formation of *Āma*

The process of digestion and metabolism, according to Ayurveda, is dependent on *agni* (digestive fire), the most precious asset of human being. Longevity, health, vigour, strength, lustre, metabolism, immunity are all dependent on the digestive fire. Abnormal state of it leads to a diseased condition, and the totally diminished state leads to death. *Agni,* according to ancient Indian philosophies (*nyāya* and *vaiseshika*) is divided into four categories, namely:

(i) *Bhaumya* — the physical fire on earth.
(ii) *Divya* — the celestial fire like solar rays, lightening, etc.
(iii) *Audarya* — the biological fire which is responsible for digestion and metabolism.
(iv) *Ākaraja* — the fire present is metals and gems like gold, diamond, etc.

As the human body is considered as a miniature replica of the universe, the biological fire is the transformed state of physical fire and celestial fire. *Agni* (digestive fire) in the human body is responsible for digestion, combustion or oxidation, splitting, conversion, transformation, absorption, assimilation, tissue building, etc. It is believed that all internal diseases are caused by vitiation of this *agni.* There are 13 numbers of *agnis,* enumerated in Ayurveda, such as *jātharāgni*-01, *dhātvāgni*-7 and *bhutāgni*-05. *Jātharāgni* can be correlated with the digestive enzymes, secreted from the pancreas (*pachyāmānāsaya*) and small intestine (*adho-āmasaya*) and is responsible for digestion, absorption and assimilation. After the functions of *Jātharāgni, dhātvāgnis* come into play in tissue building. There are seven *dhātvāgnis,* one each for each *dhātu* (structural element), which helps in the tissue building providing nutrition to the corresponding structural element. Finally, *bhutāgnis* play their role to augment the five basic elements. Among all these, *jātharāgni* (digestive fire) is considered as the most important, corresponding to major digestion and metabolism and at the same time lending support to and augments the functions of the remaining agnis presented anywhere in the body. In Ayurveda, health and disease are dependent on nutrition that is the outcome of a perfect metabolism and later utilisation of the nutrients in tissue building under the influence of *agni* (digestive fire). Pathogenesis is the result of metabolic disturbances due to the impairment or vitiation of *agni.* Impaired and vitiated *agni* produces *āma,* the undigested or wrongly digested food particles, which behaves like a poison whether absorbed or unabsorbed. There are two types of *Āmadosha* (toxic chyme):

(1) *Apakva Annarasa Āma:* Undigested food particles that cannot be absorbed and remain in the gastrointestinal tract causing heaviness, distension, colicky pain, retention of stool and urine, indigestion, foul smelling from mouth, etc. Fasting should be done in this condition

until the toxic metabolites are expelled out through vomiting or passed out in stools.

(2) *Apakva Rasa Dhātu Āma:* These are partially digested food particles that can be absorbed, but cannot be assimilated. It is more toxic and gets lodged in the joints and structural tissues causing diseases. *Āma* (toxic metabolites) interacts with the vitiated humours (*tridosha*) and undergoes a number of biochemical reactions to yield more toxic compounds, which are the aetiological factors of a number of chronic disorders such as rheumatic arthritis, gout, atherosclerosis, skin problems, neuromuscular disorder, etc.

The causes behind the vitiation of *agni* and formation of *āma* are as follows:

(A) Dietetic causes
- (i) Overeating or eating repeatedly.
- (ii) Irregular eating patterns.
- (iii) Eating in indigestion.
- (iv) Ingestion of:
  - (a) Unwholesome food.
  - (b) Incompatible food.
  - (c) Heavy and indigestible food.
  - (d) Putrid or infected food.
  - (e) Cold and stale food.
  - (f) Dry, dirty, old and unbalanced food.
- (v) Doing exercise or any strenuous work after taking meal.

(B) Abnormal seasons.

(C) Volitional suppression of natural urges.

(D) Iatrogenic factors like:
- (i) Inappropriate administration of medicines.
- (ii) Adverse effects of therapeutic measures like emesis, purgation, enema, etc.

(E) Influence of emotional states like:
- (i) Lust.
- (ii) Anger.

(iii) Greediness.
(iv) Enviness, enmity.
(v) Impatience.
(vi) Crying or pessimistic attitude.
(vii) Fear complex.

Due to above aetiological factors, the three humours get vitiated and influence the *agni* (digestive fire) to get vitiated. There are four states of *agni*, depending upon the dominant influences of the three humours. These are:

(1) ***Vishama*: Irregular due to *vāta* predominance**
A person with irregular digestive power has a perfect digestion sometimes but at other times suffers from indigestion, distension of abdomen, colicky pain, constipation, heaviness of limbs, diarrhoea and dysentery. Treatment should be given to pacify *vāta dosha* (humour) and increase the digestive power (*agni*).

(2) ***Tikshna*: Aggravated or sharp due *pitta* predominance**
In this condition, the digestive power is excessively sharp so that it can easily digest a heavy meal. A person with a sharp digestive power has a voracious appetite and takes glutton of foods repeatedly. Still the person suffers from parched lips, throat, palate, generalised heat, weight gain and other disorders. Treatment should be given to pacify the humour *pitta* and bring down the digestive power to normal.

(3) ***Manda*: Mild or weak due to *kapha* predominance**
Due to the dominant influence of the humour *kapha*, the digestive power (*agni*) gets inhibited and becomes mild or weak. A person with a weak digestive power is unable to digest even a small quantity of food and suffers from indigestion, acidity, headache, pain, constipation, etc. Treatment should be given to pacify the kapha humour and increase the digestive power by appetisers.

(4) ***Sama*: Balanced due to the balanced state of the three humours**
When the three humours are at a state of equilibrium, the digestive fire (*agni*) remains balanced or ideal. A person with an ideal or balanced

digestive fire digests food easily and does not suffer from any gastro-intestinal disorder. He ensures a proper digestion in a proper time without any complaints. The aim of an Ayurvedic treatment is to acquire this ideal digestive fire. This is the first line of treatment in almost all the diseases in Ayurveda.

Āma (toxic chyme or toxic lymph and blood), resulting from an incomplete and improper digestion, interacts with the vitiated humours (*tridosha* — *vāta*, *pitta* and *kapha*) and the combination gives rise to a number of acute and chronic diseases. *Āma* is a heavy unctuous, viscid, foul smelling, toxic fluid. Generalised symptoms of an *āma* affected disorder are indigestion, weakness, obstruction of transporting channels, improper functioning of the heart, liver and kidney, laziness, drowsiness, heaviness in stomach and limbs, anorexia, retention of stool and urine, expectoration, etc. The distinguished signs are coated tongue, slow, weak and heavy pulse, foul smelling of stool and urine with varying colours, urine with high specific gravity, etc.

When *āma* is produced as a result of incomplete and improper digestion, the process of tissue building becomes a "flaw". Toxic metabolites lodge in the tissues and joints and exhibit abnormal toxic symptoms. The unhealthy tissues, thus formed, lead to the retention of toxins. The accumulated toxins produce the disease and spread all over the body to affect other healthy tissues.

Treatment of āma conditions

Fasting is the best method for treating different stages of *āma* affected disorders. In the initial or acute stages of *āma*, one should undertake fasting till *āma* gets digested i.e. when the symptoms of *āma* or indigestion disappear and one feels light. The administration of medicines is contraindicated at this stage; however, digestive medicines or appetisers can be administered. In case of retention of toxic food materials in the stomach, emesis or gastric lavage should be done. As a consequence of indigestion or food poisoning, if diarrhoea or vomiting occurs, the physician should not stop it because it may lead to retention of toxins. In case of *āma* or toxins accumulated in tissues and spreading all over the body, medicines should be prescribed to expel them out. *Pancakarma* (five therapeutic measures) treatment is very useful in these conditions. Ingestion of medicated ghee is prescribed along with external oleation and sweating to make the toxins soft and movable. In this process, the toxins are brought to the gastrointestinal tract, from where they are expelled out by administration of emesis, purgation and enema. Appetisers and digestives are also prescribed to digest small amounts of toxins accumulated in the tissues.

3.5 Pathogenesis in Ayurveda

Pathogenesis provides the knowledge regarding the development of a disease starting from aetiology to appearance of signs and symptoms and later complications. Ayurveda describes pathogenesis of a disease in six stages and advocates the treatment to be implemented at earlier stages so that the pathogenesis cannot be evolved as a fullgrown disease. Ancient adepts of Ayurveda visualise pathogenesis at molecular level even at the start of incubation period and advise to start the treatment as soon as possible, aiming at the root causes. As the pathogenesis progresses, the disease evolves slowly and becomes full grown with complete signs and symptoms, which is described as the fifth stage in Ayurveda. The last stage is the stage of complications. Each stage of pathogenesis is suitable for treatment if the physician is able to recognise the condition and is termed as *kriyākāla* i.e. time period for treatment. However, in conventional medicine, doctors treat the patient with a state of completely evolved disease or even with late complications. Sometimes, they only suppress the symptoms but are unable to eradicate the disease because at the time when the patient comes to a doctor, the disease has been developed fully causing tissue derangement and organic dysfunction. To ensure a complete cure, it is very essential to start the treatment at the earlier stages of pathogenesis much before the organic dysfunction or tissue degeneration. Therefore, Ayurveda divides the pathogenesis into six stages with distinct signs and symptoms and describes the principles of treatment for these conditions. The six stages of pathogenesis are:

(1) **Stage of accumulation (*Samcayāvasthā*)**
Due to the intake and practice of various aetiological factors, the humours get vitiated and accumulated either locally or at their major

sites. For example, vitiated *vāta* accumulates in the rectum and large intestine, while vitiated *pitta* and *kapha* accumulate in the small intestine and stomach or lungs, respectively. The accumulated toxins remain dormant as they are not powerful yet to create the disease. When the accumulated toxins are triggered by more powerful dietetic and behavioural aetiologies, they get aggravated and the pathogenesis proceeds to the second stage. If the toxins are pacified or expelled out in this stage of accumulation, then there would be no further development of the disease process.

The signs and symptoms of *vāta* accumulation are fullness of stomach and gastrointestinal tract. In case of *pitta* accumulation, there will be yellowish discolouration of skin, sclera, nails, etc. and in *kapha* accumulation, there will be weak digestive fire, anorexia, heaviness of body and laziness. If the amount of toxins is small, then mild to moderate fasting is beneficial. But, if the toxins are in moderate quantity, then appetisers and digestives should be prescribed. In case of large quantities of toxins, purification of the body should be done by pancakarma procedures like emesis, purgation, enema, bloodletting, etc.

(2) Stage of aggravation (*Prakopāvasthā*)

If the accumulated toxins are not pacified or expelled out and the intake of aetiological factors continues, then the toxins get aggravated at their principal sites.

The signs and symptoms of *vāta* aggravation are abdominal pain, and movement of gases. In case of pitta aggravation, the symptoms are regurgitation with sour taste in the mouth, thirst and burning sensation. In *kapha* aggravation, the symptoms are anorexia (aversion to food), nausea, etc. Treatment should be given at this stage otherwise the aggravated humours will proceed to the third stage.

(3) Stage of dissemination (spreading) (*Prasarāvasthā*)

In this stage, the aggravated toxins spread in the body from the site of aggravation. As compared to the previous two stages, the symptoms are more generalised.

The symptoms arising due to *vāta* are opposite movements of gases, tympanitis with gurgling sound in abdomen, etc. The symptoms due to pitta dissemination are localised burning sensation, generalised burning sensation, asphyxiation feeling, etc. Spreading of *kapha* humour gives rise to symptoms like anorexia, indigestion, body ache and vomiting. At this stage, there is yet no involvement of body tissues or organs.

(4) **Stage of localisation of toxins (*Sthānasamsrayāvasthā*)**
If treatment is not done even at the stage of dissemination, the toxins get localised in the site, where the disease is supposed to be created. There is tissue or organic involvement at this stage and slight dysfunction is manifested. At this stage, prodromal symptoms of the disease appear, due to slight affection of the involved tissues or organ and localised toxins. This stage is also called as the stage of prodromal symptoms. It is more important than the previous three stages because the prodromal symptoms are clear indicative of the disease. Yet, manifestation of the disease can still be prevented by administering proper treatment. The prodromal symptoms may be general or specific depending upon the tissue or organ involved. In Ayurveda, specific prodromal signs and symptoms are described for each disease along with suitable treatments. If the physician is able to distinguish the prodromal signs and symptoms and starts the treatment immediately, then he would be successful in preventing more tissue or organ involvement and thus ensures a complete cure.

(5) **The stage of full blown disease (*Vyaktāvasthā*)**
If treatment is not given even in the stage of prodromal symptoms, the disease manifests and the classical signs and symptoms of the disease become apparent. This stage signifies that the involved tissues or organs are overpowered by the toxins and the body defence mechanism fails to control it. The clinical manifestations of the disease offer important information regarding the diagnosis, differential diagnosis, prognosis and treatment. This is the last stage for treating the patient, failing which complications would arise with organic dysfunctions and tissue derangements.

(6) **Stage of complications (*Bhedāvasthā*)**
If treatment is not done even in the stage of full blown disease, complications arise. In this stage, the disease becomes more difficult to

cure and sometimes becomes chronic or incurable. The complications are due to tissue derangements or organic dysfunctions. Although the symptoms can be suppressed, there would be no complete cure to the disease. To ensure a complete cure, it is highly essential to start the treatment at an earlier stage of pathogenesis.

3.6 *Three Sites of Disease* (*Traya Rogamārga*)

The diseases can be categorised into three sites of involvement depending upon their mode of transmission and site of manifestation. They are:

(1) **Outer Sites (*Bāhya Rogamārga*):** These include the skin and the structural elements (*dhātus*) except lymphatic tissues. Diseases like goitre, cellulites, skin diseases, piles, abscess, erysipelas, mole, cyst, papilloma of skin, etc. occur in these sites.
(2) **Middle Sites (*Madhyama Rogamārga*):** These include the vital points, joints, ligaments, nerves and tendons. The diseases are paralysis, paraplegia, Bell's palsy, tuberculosis, and diseases of heart, brain, kidneys and urinary bladder, etc.
(3) **Inter Sites (*Ābhyantara Rogamārga*):** These include the gastrointestinal tract and abdomen. Diseases occurring in these sites are fever, diarrhoea, vomiting, cholera, gastroenteritis, constipation, cough, asthma, and other diseases of gastrointestinal tract.

References

Acharya, Y.T. (2001). *Ayurved Dipika Commentary of Chakrapani on Charak Samhita*, 5th Edition. Choukhambha Sanskrit Sansthan, Varanasi, India.

Shastri, A. (1997). *Ayurved Tatwa Sandipika commentary on Sushrut Samhita*, 11th Edition. Choukhambha Sanskrit Sansthan, Varanasi, India.

Tripathy, B. (1998). *Charak Chandrika Commentary on Charak Samhita*, 5th Edition. Chowkhamba Surbharti Prakashan, Varanasi, India.

Tripathy, B. (2003). *Nirmala Hindi Commentary on Astanga Hridaya*, 1st Edition. Chowkhambha Sanskrit Pratisthan, Delhi, India.

Chapter 4

Chinese Medicine: Principles on Health and Diseases

Ping-Chung Leung

Abstract

Traditional Chinese Medicine (TCM) has been systematised in practice and developed many methods to maintain health during thousands of years. It is a unique philosophical system that holds a view about human health different from that of modern medicine today. Good health is the result of a comprehensive approach of maintaining the physiological harmony within the body and between the individual and the environment. These mutual relationships and principles apply to the treatment and prevention of disease, and health maintenance.

Keywords: Traditional Chinese Medicine; Principles; Theoretical Concepts; Health.

4.1 Introduction

Traditional Chinese Medicine (TCM) is built on a unique system of theoretical concepts. The theories provide a framework related to health and diseases, the normal healthy situations and the abnormal occurrences, and the relationship between what is happening within the human body and what is being manifested and felt. The understanding about health and diseases is not built on knowledge about body structures or pathological causes. Instead, diagnoses are made according to syndrome (a group of symptoms) analysis and the treatment that follows is based on the syndrome as well as an inner feeling from both patient and clinician, of the disharmony between the physiological forces within the patient.

4.2 Philosophical Backing

The most important theory that governs Chinese medicine is that of holism. The human body exists as an organic entity, which although composed of different tissues and organs, functions as a whole. Apparently, individual units are closely linked, influencing one another intimately. Holism extends beyond the human to the outside environment which directly and indirectly affects, positively or negatively influences the individual. Manifestations of pathological events might be centralised on certain organs or tissues and reflected as such; however, the attending clinician should keep a holistic mind and not be biased.

The philosophy of holism extends to the relationship between the individual and nature, so that seasonal and climatic factors should not be ignored apart from essential considerations like gender, age and general physiological constitution (O'Brien and Xue, 2015).

The mental aspects, i.e. the mind, emotion and the body are seen as a continual whole, and some organs are identified as being specific for certain emotions: e.g. anger affecting liver, worry affecting spleen and oversatisfaction affecting heart.

As the complicated internal forces are interacting with one another, one single most important fundamental theory governs the overall picture: the *Yin–Yang* theory. It is a dialectic belief that all events are the results of two opposing forces, *Yin* and *Yang* (Maciocia, 1989). *Yin* and *Yang* ideally stay in good equilibrium so that physiological processes are smoothly maintained. *Yin* and *Yang* thus become mutually interdependent and collaborate with each other when transformation is required. The experienced clinician should be capable of identifying the relative state of *Yin* and *Yang* on analysing the pathophysiological situation. When the *Yin–Yang* balance is lost, the equilibrium is tilted towards either the *Yin* or *Yang* side, and it is up to the clinician to restore a balance (Cai *et al.*, 1955).

4.3 Working Principles

Under the situation that a clinician is required to serve a patient, his line of intellectual analysis would strictly follow the *Yin–Yang* logic as has been described in the section above. With the lack of knowledge about body structures, i.e. anatomy, body function, i.e. physiology and abnormal circumstantial situations, i.e. pathology, using the simple theory of *Yin* and *Yang* for the analysis of health is handy and practical. Nevertheless, the complexities of clinical manifestations obviously demand more guiding principles for more thorough deductions and treatment planning. This practical need has initiated the inclusion of another working principle, *viz.* the five elements: generative and control cycles. The five elements are wood, fire, earth, metal and water, which symbolise the fundamental qualities and behavioural patterns of the universe, hence also the human body. The generative cycle is represented by the five elements existing in harmony and the wheel turns well. When the elements are not in harmony, the inner cycle of control between the different forces starts to function (Fig. 4.1). Each internal organ in the human body is designated to one essential element so that problems happening in the organ could be

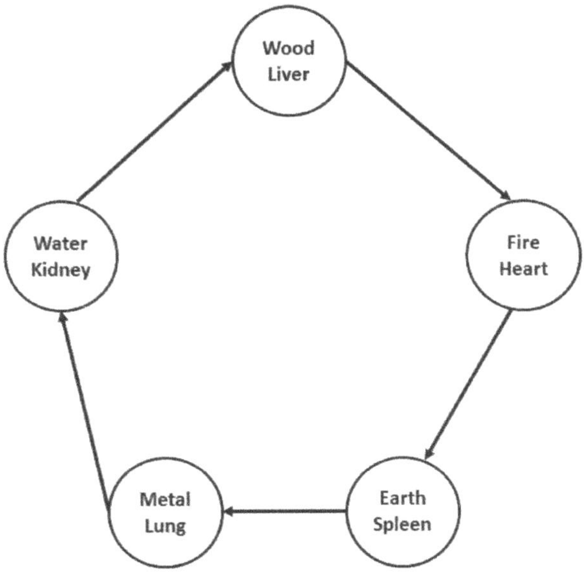

Figure 4.1. Generative cycle of five elements.

interpreted as problems related to that specific element which can be calmed or supplemented by an appropriate force in the inner cycle. On a more sophisticated level, not only organs, but physiological activities e.g. development, emotion, body fluids, excretions, etc., are correlated with the elementary forces which need to be clarified to achieve a harmony.

4.4 Diagnosis

When facing a patient, a clinical decision has to be made according to the diagnosis, which in TCM, refers to "Where" is the loss of balance, "What" is missing or excessive, and "How" does it happen. The intellectual analysis of *Yin–Yang* and the five-element cycles would require more clinical data. Acquisition of the data is achieved via a stereotyped clinical process of inspection, listening, inquiry and palpation. This classical process resembles closely the modern clinical practice in diagnosis: history taking followed by clinical examinations. Completion of data collection allows the synthesis of a syndrome, indicating the major areas of clinical concern. The experienced clinician would not be satisfied with these early results of deduction. Based on the Holistic theory, he would immediately work out the different forces that would have interacted to lead to the loss of equilibrium. In other words, what has gone wrong with the cycles of the five elements, and what are the organs responsible (Cai *et al.*, 1955; Yin and Shuai 1992).

Another set of theories is created to help defining the individual's physiological constitution that is affecting his loss of balance *viz.* the "pattern" determination which allows a logical, dynamic adjustment of treatment details. Four opposing pairs of physiological states are believed to exist in every individual, *viz. Yin/Yang*; cold/hot; superficial/deep and deficient/excessive. The existing states of the four opposing pairs, the degree of balance or imbalance would need to be defined to find out the "pattern" of the individual so that proper management can be provided. Without the appropriate consideration of the individual's "pattern", management would tend to be partial and incomplete.

Within the diagnostic observations, there is another physiological aspect that has been repeatedly stressed. It is the detection of *Qi* which is a subjective feeling of the patient and an inner feeling of the clinician about the flow of harmony or circulation of balanced body and mind. The *Qi* is very much related to the general state before and after clinical treatment.

4.5 Analysis of Diagnostic Data

As stated above, the collection of clinical data should be considered together with the general constitution, i.e. patterns, of individuals which are cross influential with each other.

The collected data are expected to allow a better understanding of the causation of the syndrome being manifested. When causation is related to climatic change or outside environment, management should follow accordingly. It is much emphasised that syndrome manifestations could be related to emotional disturbances which directly affect the *Qi*, stagnation of which leads to circulatory upsets and phlegm production. Planning of management based on syndrome observation would also consider the diet, physical and sexual activities.

With regard to chronic presentations, internal causes are considered most important. Thus, internal organs are considered individually as well as jointly in the search for evidences of interconnected disturbances. Interventions would follow the inner circle control of the five elements. Particular emotional states may be caused by dysfunction of particular organs. For example, the heart is the most important of organs that takes care of the individual's spirit, mind and emotions, hence is also responsible for the maintenance of *Qi* which should be protected at all cost (Birch and Cuadros, 2014).

In cases that the syndrome manifested fails to illustrate neither the causative mechanism nor the particular organs involved, Chinese medicine clinician would simply rely on a broad interpretation relevant to the situation of *Qi*. The clinician is always capable of defining whether it is an "excess" type of disorder or "deficient" type affecting the *Qi* at fault.

The basic concept about *Qi* is both materialistic and functional. In the material sense, it refers to a vital energy within the body responsible for the physiological functions (Cheng, 1987). *Qi*, together with body fluids, contributes towards blood circulation. In the functional sense, *Qi* is a reflection of the activities of the vital organs (Yin and Shuai, 1992; Cheng, 1987).

Qi circulates through the body along the meridians, hence can be understood as being responsible for the body energy. *Qi* is required for growth, regeneration and vitalization. *Qi* is also essential for regulatory functions and adaptations. Indications of a deficiency of *Qi* could be very obvious when there is a gross loss of energy, shortness of breath, sweating, weak voice, poor sleep and susceptibility to ailments. On the other hand, early deficiency could be very subtle and is only felt by the individual. *Qi* is difficult for diagnosis. Yet *Qi* readily gives guidance to management.

4.6 Management — Treatment

After a thorough analysis of the manifestations of a complex syndrome, the location of the imbalance and the likely internal organs involved would become clear to the clinician. Whether the problems are related to external or internal causes could also be worked out. Based on a careful scrutiny of the state of *Qi* and the general physiological constitution (pattern) of the patient, an appropriate plan of management action to counteract the deficiency or excesses could be worked out. Unlike modern hospital medicine, the management usually does not involve direct targets. Instead, symptom control and balancing policies will be adopted. Thus, in cancer treatment for example, the plan would not be a direct removal of the pathology, but a management plan to maintain survival and a reasonable quality of life. For allergies, it would be counteracting heat and dampness. For bone and joint pathologies, it would be maintenance of renal well-being, etc. Elevating the usually low level *Qi* is most likely included in the treatment plan.

Addressing the imbalance is always emphasised and the practice always involves the prevention of deterioration. Even before the manifestation of symptoms, prevention needs to be started. In modern medicine, prevention refers to public health issues: environmental hygiene, vaccinations, etc. In TCM, the emphasis is on personal care. The individual should be responsible for his own well-being. Maintain a good physiological balance through body training, keeping healthy lifestyles and careful with dietary choices. The individual should have the awareness of adverse affections, and before the actual symptoms are developed and felt, he should be alert on their prevention and try his best on the practice of "treating before the disease comes" (Ross, 1985).

4.7 Conclusion

In conclusion, TCM is a unique philosophical system that holds a view about human health different from that of modern medicine today. It takes a view that good health is the result of a comprehensive approach of maintaining the physiological harmony within the body and between the individual and the environment. Treatment aims at the control of symptoms as well as correcting the loss of harmony within the human body. Most importantly, individuals should be responsible for their own well-being and healthy existence and actively resist the loss of bodily harmony.

References

Birch, S. and Cuadros, M.R. (2014). *Restoring Order in Health and Chinese Medicine Studies of the Development of Qi and the Channels.* La Liebre de Marzo, Barcelona.

Cai, G., Chao, G. and Chen, D. (1955). *Advanced Textbook on Traditional Chinese Medicine and Pharmacology*, Vol. 1. New World Press, Beijing.

Cheng, X. (1987). *Chinese Acupuncture and Moxibustion.* Foreign Language Press, Beijing.

Maciocia, G. (1989). *The Foundations of Chinese Medicine: A Comprehensive Text for Acupuncturists and Herbalists.* Churchill Livingstone, New York.

O'Brien, K.A. and Xue, C.C. (2015). The theoretical framework of Chinese medicine. In: *A Comprehensive Guide to Chinese Medicine.* World Scientific Publisher, Singapore.

Ross, J. (1985). *Zang Fu — The Organ Systems of Traditional Chinese Medicine*, 2nd Edition. Churchill Livingston, Edinburgh.

Yin, H.H. and Shuai, H.C. (1992). *Fundamentals of Traditional Chinese Medicine.* Foreign Language Press, Beijing.

Chapter 5

Research and Development of Chinese Medicinal Plants

Clara Bik-San Lau, Erik Chun-Hay Ko, Johnny Chi-Man Koon, Grace Gar-Lee Yue and Ping-Chung Leung

Abstract

Traditional medicine (TM) has taken care of people's health in China for 3,000 years. With the many successes in the past of drug discovery from botanical origins, the popular use of proprietary herbal drug and with the rising popularity of health supplements, medicinal herbs should have a bright future for better and more innovative developments. The strong historical background and the rich collections of classical records on the clinical uses of herbs in Chinese medicine should adequately encourage strong commitments from both academic and industrial sectors.

Keywords: Chinese Medicinal Plants; Evidence-Based Health Supplements; Drug Discovery; Functional Food; Innovative Developments.

5.1 Introduction

Chinese medicine has a long history of over 3,000 years. With China's large size and active commercial activities across its neighbouring countries and states, not only the original medicinal material and practices are plentiful, but also others which were not original to China Mainland have been brought in. Thus, Chinese medicine, since hundreds of years ago, has been an amalgamation of health practices of multiple origins: south west from the Indians, west from the Persians, possibly Egyptians and Greeks, and north from the Mongols and Koreans (Fu, 1985; Huard and Wong, 1968).

Like all health and medical practices, small-scale native traditions serving specific needs are the initiating forces before larger scale and generalised applications start. In the process of wider, general applications, scholars and the imperial court get involved. The Taoists, Buddhists and Confucians in China, therefore, are not only housekeepers of Chinese Medicine at different stages, but have given a lot of inventional ideas escorting its gradual maturation and further development (McGrew, 1985; Beinfield and Korngold, 1991; Feng and Tsu, 1972). Unlike India, the neighbour, which allowed extremely strong religious and possibly superstitious leadership in the form of Ayurveda, Yogic and Tantric medical practices, the influence of Taoists, Confucians, and Buddhists remains philosophical. Apparently, both healers and philosophers agree to allow an obvious boundary to exist between practice and thinking, both of which, however, reach some sort of integration under practical circumstances (Jaggi, 1981; Takakusu, 1956; Heyn, 1987).

Traditional medicine (TM) has taken care of people's health in China for 3,000 years; not until 150 years ago in the Qing Dynasty when European missionaries brought in allopathic medicine with the whole system of structural explanations (i.e. anatomy), together with the physiological and pathological mysteries, later the fascinating varieties of treatment, that Chinese people were awaken, after a period of amazement, that modern advances could offer so much more, on top of the traditional practice.

One major difference between traditional and modern allopathic medicine is that allopathic medicine is reductionistic, aiming at the identification of a problem which is subsequently removed. When the target problem is clear, exists singly and is removable, the outcome could be highly impressive. However, when the problem could be multiple, complex or not removable, The solution could only be partial or compromising (Leung, 2001; Kaptchuk and Eisenberg, 1998; Fair, 1999).

In spite of the tremendous advances in allopathic medicine, and many apparently desperate problems have been solved using modern technology and scientific methods and devices, some complicated pathological problems remain irremovable. Common examples of pathologies that disappoint not only the patients but also threaten the Public Health Authorities are viral infections, aging and aging related diseases, allergies and cancers. Decades of research concentrating on single targets and immediate relieves have led to successes as well as disappointments, so that it is now realised that the allopathic approach to pathological problems could be reaching its limit when many of such problems are not of simple but of complex nature, so that a single potent agent, would fail to offer the relief. When a number of supportive measures are jointly used, the chance could be much better. Very often, the outcome of the multiple attempts is the maintenance of the individual's physiological balance.

With the realisation of this new therapeutic logic, Chinese medicine, which has its emphasis on the harmonisation of physiological balance, would enjoy new attention. The traditional practice does not master the knowledge of complicated pathological changes leading to syndromes of suffering. The practice thus only helps by calming down the syndrome of sufferings through multiple efforts to harmonise the disturbances at various levels. Such approach is naturally slow and accumulative, thus never comparable to interventions using sharp, aggressive therapies routinely administered in allopathic medical practice of today (Lai, 2001; Tang and Eisenberg, 1992).

5.2 Practice of Chinese Medicine in China and Chinese Community

While allopathic medicine is really reaching its limits and more attention is being paid on Traditional Chinese Medicine (TCM), one wonders, whether in China and in other Chinese Communities, TCM is gaining increasing popularity.

Since there is a current need for a medical service that could supplement the deficient practice of allopathic medicine which might be described as possibly too specific, and that maintenance of physiological balances is equally important, Chinese medicine in China and Chinese Communities would be a timely offer. It is therefore appropriate to give a careful scrutiny on the situation of Chinese medicine in China and

Chinese Communities. Special attention should be focused on whether the traditional practice has followed the steps of modernisation.

TCM service in China is being offered in hospitals called "Chinese medicine hospitals" or Chinese medicine Clinics. In fact, the so-called "Chinese medicine hospitals" are just like any hospital offering comprehensive varieties of specialties: internal medicine, surgery, obstetrics, paediatrics, etc. Only that herbal treatment is more freely available. In fact, in all hospitals in China, TCM service is available on patients' requests. Traditional practitioners have been complaining that there has been too much "westernisation" in their stream of practice. The sad things is hospitalised patients are given more allopathic drugs than Chinese medicine. The outpatient clinics, on the other hand, are crowded with patients demanding acupuncture, manipulations and other quick manual therapies. Education for the production of qualified practitioners consists of two separate streams, *viz.* modern and traditional practice. However, the young graduates who are free to follow either modern or traditional practice, would favour modern practices and pharmaceutical prescriptions which tend to be simple and straightforward compared with the traditional practice which relies heavily on experience.

In other Chinese Communities like Hong Kong and Singapore, Modern medicine is the mainline practice while TCM mainly serves those who seek relief for ailments or become disappointed with varieties of modern treatment.

It is apparent that modern medicine has already replaced TM in China and other Chinese Communities while TCM today has not attained modernisation so that the practice is not much different from the old practices hundreds of years ago. If research is the only approach that might lead to advances, it is logical to look towards the research engagements in this traditional area to check whether it could become more capable to supplement what is needed for deficiencies in modern medicine (Leung, 2008).

5.3 Research on Chinese Medicinal Herbs in the Past Decades

Putting aside the practice of Chinese medicine, which involves many varieties of treatment, one could concentrate on the use of medicinal herbs and examine how the traditional plants could be utilised in the modern world.

The practice of TCM in Chinese Communities could be old and lacking innovation, but the value of Chinese medicinal herbs has never been ignored. Pharmaceutical companies, of course, are aware of the potential of medicinal herbs turning into potent drugs. Clinicians and herbal experts have also been creatively modifying the traditional varieties of application.

Some details of the different directions of research are given as follows:

(I) Pharmaceutical drug discovery from medicinal herbs.
(II) Proprietary drugs from medicinal herbs.
(III) Rediscovery of old herbal formulae.
(IV) Health supplements using medicinal herbs.
(V) "Fractionation cocktails" from herbal extracts.

5.3.1 *Pharmaceutical Drug Discovery from Medicinal Herbs*

Experts in the pharmaceutical industry understand that many successful drugs are in fact developed from botanical items. With the strong history of small molecules successfully discovered from plants, later proven to be potent target orientated drugs, thousands of chemists have continued to engage in never-ending discoveries. Of the many recent successes, Vincristine from periwinkle flower and Taxol from Yew Bark must be impressive examples that are earning pharmaceutical companies trillions of dollars. Both Taxol and Vincristine are successful examples of the Phytochemistry division of the National Centre for Scientific Research of France (CNRS) at Gif which has strong commitments on tropical plants screening for the purpose of drug discovery. In China, the antimalarial drug Artemisinin was developed from Qinghao, a Chinese herbal classic used for malignant fever. Although the Chinese chemist responsible for its chemical refinement does not own any patent, her contribution has earned her significant recognition and praises (Tu, 2011; Boik, 1996).

The story of discovery of Artemisinin from the Chinese medicinal herb Qinghao is interesting. Dr. Y.Y. Tu was a young scientist assigned to lead a Malaria research group in a National Campaign against Malaria.

The team consisted of phytochemists and pharmacologists. They screened 2,000 Chinese herbs and identified 640 that had possibly anti-malarial activities. A mouse model of malaria was used for proper evaluation. An extract of *Artemisia annua* showed a promising degree of inhibition against parasite growth but this observation was not reproducible in subsequent experiments. Tu re-examined carefully the ancient records and found that when Qinghao extract was used for malignant fever, the plant was not boiled to high temperatures. Tu's group thence used low temperature extractions and obtained much better biological activities in the malaria model. What followed was the gradual chemical analysis of the Chemical structure of Artemisinin.

It is envisaged that many other traditional Chinese herbs should contain chemicals responsible for their recorded clinical activities. The logical deduction from the Qinghao discovery has driven thousands of scientists in China to join the quest for new drugs to be isolated from medicinal herbs.

Pharmaceutical development from medicinal herbs is time consuming and resource dependent. The enthusiasm undoubtedly will continue. Many available plants, particularly those with historical records of specific efficacies, will be explored repeatedly and their extract derived small molecules will be tested against specific biological targets. Small molecule discovery is not difficult. Subjecting them to verify their therapeutic efficacies, however, will remain in the hands of major resourceful pharmaceutical industries (Crutchley *et al.*, 2010; Tatti *et al.*, 2008). Only those enterprises are capable of arranging extensive and expensive research programs that are required to allow the products to be marketed as safe and efficacious drugs.

When phytochemists successfully convert extracts of medicinal herbs into drugs, it is doubtful whether the herbs related could still be considered "Chinese medicine". This way of transforming Chinese medicine into pharmaceuticals, therefore, would not be discussed further in this review.

5.3.2 *Proprietary Drugs from Medicinal Herbs*

Traditionally, Chinese medicine is being prescribed as "formulae", i.e. combination of many items of medicinal material, based on their individual clinical properties as well as their combined effects. Guiding principles have been developed to allow the combined herbal components to reach additive or synergistic effects in order to bring about the greatest effects of symptom control. Historically, hundreds of herbal formulae have been used and recorded, together with their modifications. Different formulae have been advocated for the same group of symptoms, whereas some others are advocated only for very specific indications.

Throughout the centuries, neighbouring countries around China, notably Korea and Japan, have great respect on Chinese medicine and endorsed a large number of the classical treatment formulae, as standard prescriptions for groups of syndrome presentations. Thus in Japan, since the Meiji Revolution, 210 such formulae, known as Kampo medicine, have been documented and endorsed to be prescribed in Government Hospitals (Ichiko, 2011; Watanabe *et al.*, 2001). The Korean Health Authority has the similar tradition. The largest users of herbal formulae remain to be people within China and other Chinese Communities.

Whether used exactly as their original formulation, or as Kampo in Japan, or as Oriental medicine in Korea, these classical formulations follow closely the ancient descriptions. Only minor addition or subtraction of one or a few items are allowed so as not to down value the original therapeutic effects. The indications are all well-known although the herbal clinician could give limited adjustments for special reasons. The attitude of both users and recipients maintain a fervent trust on the herbal formulae which they believe would facilitate good outcomes.

This is a clear demonstration of the triumph of the tradition. The users are not demanding any change in the old contents. Kampo in Japan and Oriental formulations in Korea have adopted the same treatment philosophy. They have solid trust on the tradition and never doubt the efficacy of the formulae. For them, modern update justification is not necessary. Safety and efficacy are believed to have been secured already in the long years of successful applications and patient safety. With this background, the traditional herbal formulae have enjoyed quite steady markets and remained popular either as prescribed items among herbal clinicians or as patient self-administered symptom control treatment choices among the users who prefer not to rely on medical consultations when facing health hazards and ailments (Watanabe, 2007; Taira *et al.*, 2004; Itoh *et al.*, 2002; Nagano *et al.*, 1999).

Kampo medicine in Japan is based on ancient Chinese medicinal formulae that have acquired not only persistent trust among the users but the Japanese Health Authority is also energetically supporting its research. The major areas of research interest included herb safety, herbs for Cancer treatment, marine medicinal herbs and infection control (Watanabe *et al.*, 2011).

The ministry of Health, Labour and Welfare in Japan has endorsed 210 Kampo formulae which could be prescribed for any patient under national insurance cover. An official list of Kampo medicine is available in its official website. Information ranges from single herbs, Kampo formulae, extracts, preparations, origins of supply, ingredients, etc. (JP14, 2002).

The World Health Organization (WHO) believes that it is highly justified to promote TM as important contributing components in the delivery of primary health care. It has given a strong message that the centuries of safe and effective utilisations could be considered strong evidences of safety and essential efficacy which would allow further research using modern scientific methodologies (WHO, 2000; Goldbeck-Wood and Dorozynski, 1996; Campion, 1993). Indeed, regulatory bodies in the world would agree with WHO's recommendation today (FDA, US & SFDA, China). The proprietary formulae therefore, are entering a new era of development, which will lead to better understanding of the indications and mechanisms of action, with and without modifications (Eisenberg *et al.*, 1993; Cheng, 2003; Traditional Medicine EDM, 2002).

Old formulae could have related or divergent indications which are all well recorded. Today's users in China, Japan and Korea tend to closely follow the classical recommendations. The users are free to choose the formula of his taste for particular indications of his choice. The producers stick to the details of the contents in the production of the old formula and are competitive only on the quality control (QC) and packaging. Innovations related to proprietary formulations, therefore, are quite limited.

5.3.3 *Rediscovery of Old Herbal Formulae*

Drug discovery in modern pharmaceuticals starts from the identification of small chemical molecules, followed by subjecting them to biological research platforms to work out their mechanisms of action. The same research platforms could be applied to the study of single herb extracts or herbal formulae. The revelation of biological effects of single herbs and mixtures has initiated innovative explorations on the specific uses of classical herbs and classical herbal formulae.

Thus, the research platforms have been used for the better understanding of the old herbal formulae, particularly in the direction of new clinical indications and pharmacological mechanisms of action. The most conventional clinician in TCM might not care much about how modern pharmacological theory could be applied to explain the outcome of treatment and remain happy with just personal and past experience. However, young graduates of TCM have acquired sound knowledge on human physiology and pathology which would inadvertently lead them on a serious course of fact finding pursue. Enthusiasts are engaged in innovative explorations on the clinical uses of herbs, and good examples are given in the following paragraphs to demonstrate the different approaches and the future potentials.

(i) *Expansion of known clinical indications*

Many popular old formulae used by clinicians of either traditional or modern practitioners have been applied in new needy areas of symptom control. A large number of clinical reports are available in Chinese language about the effectiveness of old formulae used for the control of difficult symptoms and syndromes which might be different from classical descriptions. Kampo clinicians in Japan have widely used herbal formulae for the control of pain, sleep disorders and post-operative problems (Itoh *et al.*, 2002; Terauchi *et al.*, 2011; Manabe *et al.*, 2010; Wood *et al.*, 2010; Endo *et al.*, 2006; Kono *et al.*, 2009). The colourful clinical reports of modern applications of the old formulae do not add much pharmacological science to the old practice apart from giving it more colourful practical values.

Japanese clinicians have the tradition of using Kampo medicine to supplement modern treatment. Bowel stagnation is a common post-operative complication that endangers surgical results and unnecessarily slows down recovery. Surgeons have been engaged in clinical and bench research on a popular Kampo formula named *Dai-kenchu-to*, which is in fact a TCM formula commonly used for balancing digestion. Many reports in Japan have endorsed the efficacy of this herbal preparation for the treatment of post-operative ileus (Endo *et al.*, 2006; Iwai *et al.*, 2007) and platform studies have worked out some pharmacological channels of action (Shibata *et al.*, 1999) Kono, Professor in Surgery from the Nagasaki University in 2009, strongly expressed his support for the use of Kampo medicine in gastroenterology (Kono *et al.*, 2008, 2009).

At least one quarter of the officially endorsed Kampo preparations are popular ancient Chinese medicine formulae. Producers are making clear general instructions for their Clinical uses. However, it is up to the users and prescribers to make innovative modifications like what the Surgeons have done for *Dai-kenchu-to*. The modifications are interesting and practical, but might be challenged for being subjective and not sufficiently supported by research. One ten-herb formula, known in Kampo as *Juzen-taiho-to*, for instance, has been advocated for boosting energy, physical strengthening, anaemia, cancer treatment and disease prevention (Kono *et al.*, 2009). The situation in China, with reference to the ancient Chinese medicine formulae, follows the same confusing direction. The need for serious research on these popular herbal formulae is therefore obvious.

(ii) *Research on specific indications*

Difficult problems exist in day-to-day clinical practices that do not find easy solutions. The traditional practice therefore might have special offers. For example, cancer treatment using cytotoxic drugs commonly leads to adverse effects like gastrointestinal symptoms of diarrhoea, nausea and vomiting. Using Chinese medicine formula to help alleviating the symptoms is already a common practice in Chinese Communities and Japan. Cheng from Yale University USA, wanted to follow a proper research system and has started an extensive study to evaluate the pharmacological effects of a classical 4 herbs formula *Huang Qin Tang* on its soothing effects on the gastrointestinal complications during cytotoxic treatment.

A comprehensive system of research to thoroughly explore the value of this herbal formula would consist of the establishment of a reliable method of QC, an unveiling of the biological mechanisms of action and finally, clinical evidences. Cheng made impressive demonstrations on all three areas of research requirements.

QC is essential to determining the consistency of botanical ingredients and to the final manufacture of botanical drugs. While rigorous clinical studies can address botanical drug safety and efficacy, there are no well accepted, modern standard for performing botanical drug QC. Current mainstream QC methods rely on technologies of the 1970s and focus on monitoring a few marker chemical compounds and/or single enzyme/receptor bioactivities. This approach, however, is inadequate in addressing the inherent complexity of botanical extracts that can contain tens or even hundreds of phytochemicals.

For botanical medicine to truly succeed, the adoption of a new, high-level standardised platform for assuring QC is crucial. The hallmarks of a modern platform for botanical drugs should include: (1) comprehensive, molecular resolution chemical fingerprints with identification of as many of the individual phytochemical constituents as possible; (2) comprehensive, sensitive bio response fingerprint; (3) statistical and quantifiable score function to define similarity of these patterns; (4) robust, reproducible and cost effective protocol for industrial use and (5) integrated informatics database for sample tracking data storage and data analysis. Such a platform has to assure both the regulatory agencies and the public that the botanical drug is manufactured to standards that are consistent over time.

QC could be further ensured using Genomic Bio response Profiling. While LC/MS represents one of the most powerful chemical analysis methodologies, there is no single analysis system that is capable of detecting every type of phytochemical compound. Hence, a separate and orthogonal methodology is required that complements the strengths of chemical characterisation. A powerful and novel platform needs to characterise not only the phytochemical compound pattern but the resulting biological response to this collection of phytochemicals.

Using a living human cell line and the genomic response transcription profile (transcriptome) as a sensitive detector, one can define an objective, unique subset of the expressed genes that defines a signature QC pattern for each botanical. Atypical signature set will involve between 20 and 40 genes that be developed into a routine plate-based quantitative real time-PCR (qRT-PCR) assay. Analysis of the expression profiles of different herbal formulations demonstrate that the response genes that are differentially expressed form a unique and quantitative set of each of the botanicals.

This bio response gene pattern can be quantified and statistically compared (Rockwell *et al.*, 2013).

It was on these biological platforms that the four-herb formula was tested for its essential biological effects as well as the molecular targets (Wang *et al.*, 2011). On the clinical side, a phase 1/2 trial was on going.

Not only was the formula found effective in diarrhoea control, but the cytotoxic effects of the drug treatment were also observed to be enhanced (Liu and Cheng, 2012; Lam *et al.*, 2010b; Wang *et al.*, 2011; Law *et al.*, 2009). This must be the first report on the double value of an old classic herbal formula during its modern application for a specific clinical purpose. The research is still going on and is expected to give further information on the clinical value.

(iii) *New innovations to verify the clinical efficacy of traditional herbal formula*

Although drug discovery in the pharmaceutical world have been very successful in the past century, in recent years, serious challenges are being met. One major cause is that there are yet no satisfactory solutions for multifactorial complex chronic diseases. Some chemical drugs proven effective for a given target have been reported to have severe side effects and are removed from market. In the pharmaceutical industry, interests on the development of multicomponent drugs have started. The logic is based on the combination of existing drugs with already known targets. The assessment for efficacy therefore would need a systems approach, analysing the complex changes in the total physiological environment.

Chinese medicine using mainly herbs in combination for health derangements is based on a systemic theory derived from long-term clinical observations. The philosophy of holism and systematology emphasises on the importance of harmony within the body and between the body and its immediate environment. The maintenance of this balance is considered more important than the simple inhibitory effects against a specific disease target. This old concept of health and disease fits well into the post-genome era of systems biology.

Systems biology recalls the ideas of holism, systematology and network. A comprehensive approach to investigate the effects of a drug item would need to be directed at the whole body system level, *viz.* the level of genes, proteins and metabolites. How the systems change in reaction to the administration of a drug item will give a true story of its effects towards the important task of maintaining the physiological harmony/balance of the body. The single target-based drug could be developed into a drug system of composite medicine that needs to be analysed at the relevant levels according to the constitutional complexity (Li *et al.*, 2002; Luo *et al.*, 2012; Luo and Wang, 1997, 1999).

With this recent development of a much more complex requirement in drug discovery, the traditional way of health maintenance and disease combat like Chinese medicine finds new aspirations. The whole responses of the body system, expressed at the levels of genes, proteins and metabolites need to be understood. The genomics, proteomics and metabolomics of the body in response to a drug system constitute the new way of exploration common to modern and tradition medicine. The systems approach studies may be used to (i) harmonise the different diagnostic systems of Chinese medicine and modern medicine and (ii) provide an integrative biomarker indicator system for the study of the physiological effects of a drug item (either chemical or herbal) under different bodily conditions.

The fundamental symptoms and signs essential for modern diagnostic and therapeutic as pathological and biochemical indicators will need to be cross checked with the data within the network of genes, proteins and the metabolites, resulting in a better characterisation of a complex disease and its responses to intervention (Hood, 1998).

Using the systems approach, popular classic herbal formulae that are likely to supplement difficult disease or degeneration areas could be subjected to a comprehensive evaluation, either in laboratory platforms or clinical settings. The logic of the classical combinations with their specific selection of herbs could likewise be scientifically studied (Ideker *et al.*, 2001; Nicholson *et al.*, 1999; Fiehn, 2002).

The systems approach will probably stay on a slow research level until more disappointment with the single target management might reveal the need for more effective complex remedies. In the meantime, the systems approach may bring traditional medicinal herbs to a scientific level as much respected as modern pharmaceuticals.

Different groups in China have started the system approach of research. One predictable difficulty lies in the dynamic state of the Big data. Correlations between the data and physiological changes are already complex and difficult. With the inevitable day to day dynamic changes of the data, correlations might become impossible.

(iv) *Creation of new herbal formula based on modern pharmacological knowledge*

Old herbal formulae are established on accumulated experiences. Today, clinical treatment is built on pathological need i.e. counteracting harmful pathological events. A disease condition is the result of harmful pathological activities which not only target against specific tissues and organs but also destroy the normal physiological harmony of the human body. Like modern pharmaceuticals which aim at specific targets, an innovative herbal formula can be created through the selection of a number of herbs with known biological activities to fight against specific pathological conditions (Leung, 2001; Kaptchuk and Eisenberg, 1998). TCM practitioners could have strong reasons to stick rigidly to the ancient formulae on which they have perfect trust, however, time has much changed since the creation of those formulae. With the established knowledge on pathology and pharmacology, the formulae could be re-examined to ensure the efficacy as well as safety. Moreover, the bioactive components of the herbs could also be explored to allow further development.

Two examples will be given as examples of how a small number of herbs could be chosen to form an innovative formula in an attempt to produce evidence-based biological and clinical effects.

A. *Creating an evidence-based herbal formula for cancer treatment*
The first example is a herbal formula created for cancer supplementary treatment currently under study in Hong Kong. Since cancer development involves complicated pathological processes of, for example, uncontrolled cellular proliferations, which could be the result of abnormal cellular activities, neovascularisations, and decline of host immunological defence, the herbal formula thus created is designed to take a combination of herbs known to be pro-apoptotic, anti-angiogenic and immuno-stimulant. The selected herbs could be tested individually on different relevant biological platforms, then combined to observe synergistic effects. A bone metastatic model is also created to investigate the control of metastasis to bone (Wong *et al.*, 1994, 2005; Kuo, *et al.*, 2006; Cheng and Leung, 2011). The platform research framework is given in the sketch diagrams (Figs. 5.1–5.4).

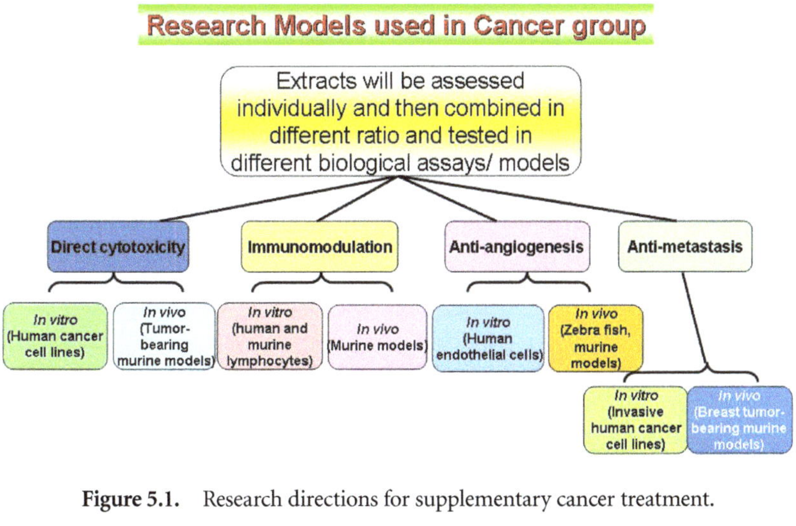

Figure 5.1. Research directions for supplementary cancer treatment.

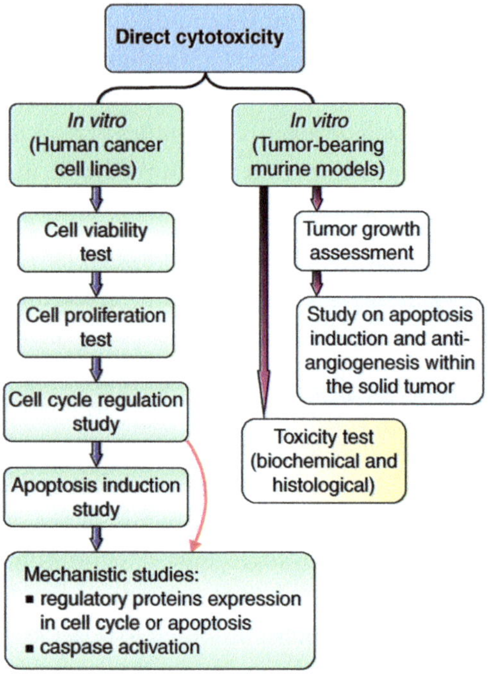

Figure 5.2. Study on direct cytotoxicity.

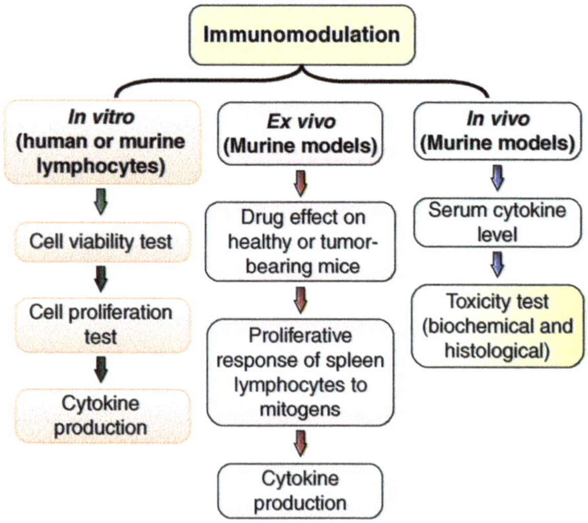

Figure 5.3. Study on immunomodulation.

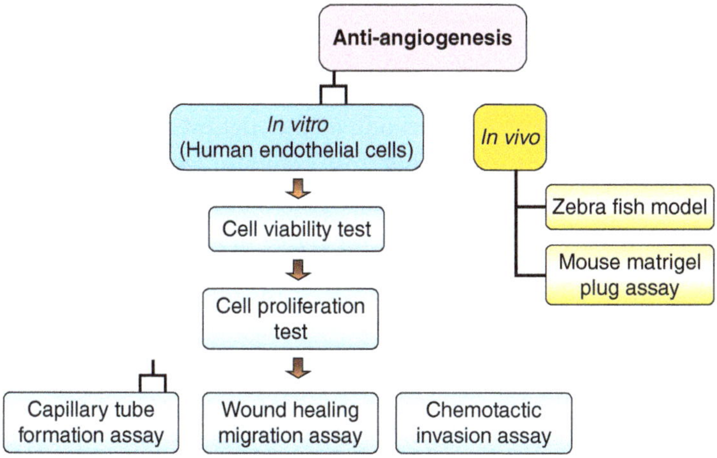

Figure 5.4. Study on anti-angiogenesis.

According to recent reports on popular herbs being used for cancer treatment in China, five herbs are chosen for platform studies. They are *Scutellaria*, *Andrographis paniculata* (for apoptosis), *Hedyotis diffusa* (for anti-angiogenetic) and *Acanthopanax senticosus*, *Ganoderma lucidum* (for immunomodulation). The herbs are studied separately for the desired bioactivities, and then combined, on *in vitro* and *in vivo* platforms.

For academic and pharmacological interests, sub-fractions are produced from different gross extracts and are tested on *in vitro* platforms to screen out those with the best biological activities. This knowledge will be important for future extension of research work. Of the five herbs used to compose the anticancer formula, three are found to be most effective in the *in vitro* studies. The two less effective herbs are thus excluded from the formulation. The three herbs selected for further study belong to the food-category of medicinal herbs that have been used on dinner tables of Chinese communities. Safety therefore is not an issue of concern. On completion of the platform studies, the formula would be put on a proper evidence-based clinical trial for cancer patients to be used as a supplement agent to maintain well-being and prevent recurrence after conventional treatment (Zhang *et al.*, 2011; Wong *et al.*, 2010; Yue *et al.*, 2011, 2012).

B. *Creating a cardiovascular protective herbal formula*

The second example is an old herbal formula to be developed into a cardiovascular tonic. Mortality arising from cardiovascular pathologies remains one of the highest. Maintenance of cardiovascular health therefore remains a universal concern. Interventional therapies and medications have made impressive advances, but preventive measures would be of equal importance. A two-herb combination created in the later part of Qing Dynasty, consisting of *Salviae Miltiorrhizae Radix et Rhizoma* and *Puerariae Lobatae Radix* is used in a combined herbal formula which has been studied extensively on cardiovascular biological platforms and then put on three clinical trials. In the laboratory, the formula was found to have the biological effects of anti-inflammation, anti-oxidation, anti-foam cell formation on vascular endothelium and vasodilation (Cheung *et al.*, 2012, 2013; Zhou *et al.*, 2012; Lam *et al.*, 2010a; Liang *et al.*, 2012; Koon *et al.*, 2011, Fong *et al.*, 2011; Ng *et al.*, 2011) (Fig. 5.5). Clinical trials using ultrasonic carotid intima thickness as a surrogate marker repeatedly showed very significant thinning benefits. No significant adverse effects were encountered.

The first randomised control trial was done for post-intervention coronary occlusion patients who were found to have two

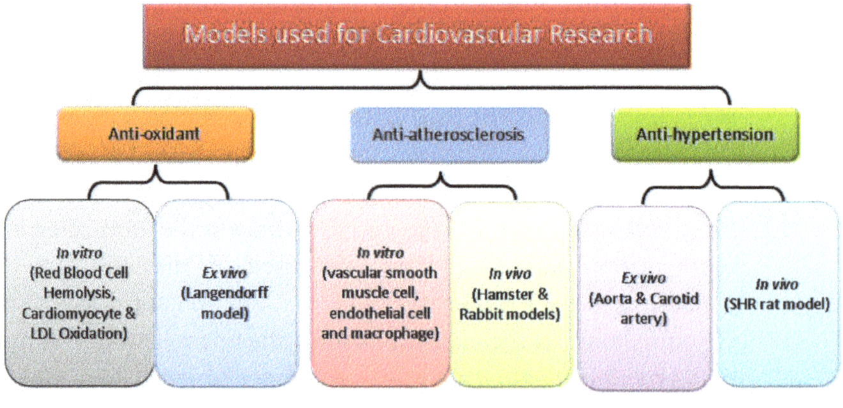

Figure 5.5. Research directions for cardiovascular protective.

coronary arteries blocked. Of the 100 patients recruited all enjoyed intima thinning of the carotid artery while the control group did not after six months of treatment. The second similarly designed control study was done for patients with diabetes and/or hypertension. Results showed 96% of the treatment group enjoying intima thinning. The third clinical trial was done for para-menopausal women who had border-line hypercholesterolemia. Again, significant thinning of the carotid intima was found in the treatment group after taking the herbal formula for 12 months.

It could therefore be recommended that the herbal formula could be used as an adjuvant therapy in cardiac patients with coronary occlusion under standard treatment or as a preventive agent among the susceptibles (Leung *et al.*, 2010, 2013; Woo *et al.*, 2013; Chan *et al.*, 2006; Koon *et al.*, 2013; Tam *et al.*, 2009).

(v) *Botanical drug product* (*FDA, USA*)

Food and Drug Administration (FDA) in the turn of the last century has set rules on the registration of a special health product, which is neither a pharmaceutical, identifiable as a small chemical molecule, nor a health supplement, which belongs to the "food" category, This new category is hence called "Botanical Drug Product". The group of chemicals contained in the Botanical Drug Product should satisfy strict QC requirements and need to go through strict clinical evaluations not much different from a proper clinical trial.

The first botanical drug product is an ointment derived from a natural product, green tea, called Veregen for the treatment of rectal and vaginal warts as a topical agent. It is a water extract of *Camellia sinensis*, containing mainly kunecatechins (85–95%), epigallocatechin, epicatechin and other catechins. The botanical drug has gone through pharmcodynamic and pharmacokinetic studies. Safety is guaranteed after randomised control studies (Tatti *et al.*, 2008). This first FDA approved botanical drug marks an important milestone in the development of Chinese medicine as the requirements to ensure the quality of the extract and its biological/clinical efficacy are excellent examples for future approvals.

The first oral botanical drug product "Crofelemer" was approved by FDA USA in 2012. "Crofelemer" is an extract from the bark of a South American plant *Croton lechleri* traditionally used by natives for the treatment of diarrhoea. Today, Crofelemer is developed for non-infections, secretory diarrhoea, e.g. among AIDS patients (Crutchley *et al.*, 2010; Tatti *et al.*, 2008; Mangel and Chaturvedi, 2008; Tradtrantip *et al.*, 2010; FDA, 2012). The chemical structure of the extract is known but some other less important components are allowed. Up to this time, it is prescribed mostly for AIDS patients while other indications like irritable bowel syndrome are being explored.

Looking at the nature of the two newly registered botanical products, many other innovations might be coming in future from medicinal plants or traditional herbal formulae. Botanical drug products will greatly enrich the armamentarium of proprietary health supporting agents.

5.3.4 *Health Supplements using Medicinal Herbs*

Health supplements include a large variety of health promoting products ranging from nutritionals like vitamins and minerals to new products of nutritional research claiming to have specific supportive effects on general health or particular physiological functions like cartilage and vascular integrities. The rising popularity has not only roused the attention of the users but the sharply increasing sales volume is sufficient to alert the producers on a competitive run. Old figures at the turn of the last century have demonstrated a national expenditure on health supplements in the US superseding the total expenses on standard primary health care (Goldbeck-Wood and Dorozynski, 1996; Eisenberg *et al.*, 1993).

Health supplements are considered extra, unimportant items for health in the modern affluent community. Health supplements in the traditional philosophy of Chinese medicine, however, have a much more important role. Dating back to the ancient times when clinical treatment was non-specific, general and untargeted, maintenance of health and prevention of falling sick was the vital aim. Traditional healers used to choose among three categories of herbs: those with known effects for longevity, those for symptom control and those for obvious life threatening conditions, to form a prescription. Herbs known to maintain longevity are considered to be of top value (Hoizey and Hoizey, 1988; Quella *et al.*, 2000). In general, health supplements, capable of preventing diseases, are considered more important than specific therapy. It is interesting to note this fundamentally different traditional philosophy as compared with modern therapeutics of today, which values only specific therapeutic effects.

Indeed, herbal medicine, as discussed earlier, covers broad target areas, acts weakly, slowly and accumulatively, in very much the same direction as health supplements. Obviously, given the very broad areas of coverage of Chinese medicine, there must be a lot to offer in the field of health supplements. We need to realise, nevertheless, in the current free market and free choices, the principles of selection.

In the last decade, the rising popularity of health supplements has persuaded the regulators to take active studies on the principles of reasonable control. The European Union has formed a large expert committee to advice on the procedures required to assess a certain health claim (PASSCLAIM) (Fig. 5.6). The related documents have since become practical guidelines (Aggett *et al.*, 2005). There are four recommended basic

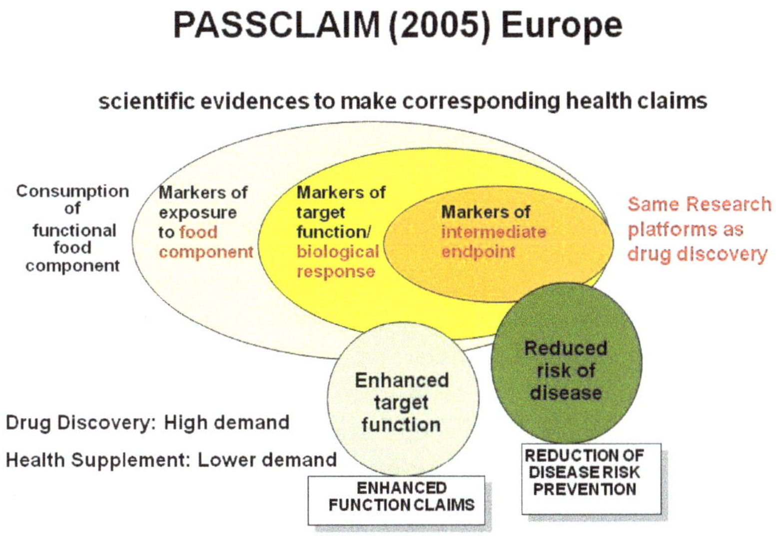

Figure 5.6. Concepts of scientific evidence and corresponding health claims.

assessment procedures before a health claim can be considered valid. Firstly, the nutritional value must be provided. Then the absorption process must be effective and efficient. Thirdly, after the intake, the metabolic assimilation and biological pathways need to be understood. Finally and most importantly, the genuine health value, in terms of disease/illness reduction and functional gains in physiological activities need to be proven.

It is therefore obvious that PASSCLAIM requires QC, mechanistic studies and clinical evaluations, very much similar to the requirements for the development of new drugs. However, there must be an acceptable compromise along the described pathway to differentiate between a health supplement from a drug. Given the yet undetermined requirements and methodology of evaluation, the assumption could be a carefully evaluated lowering of the strict standards in the final clinical evaluations (Schepetkin and Quinn, 2006; Stephens, 1999; Yang and Wang, 1993; Yun and Choi, 1998).

Looking through the rich supply of Chinese medicinal herbs that could be used as food and when the selected herbs are chosen from the "Food" category, to be used for preventive or harmonising purposes, the boundary between "treatment" and "supplement" must be quite slim. The main difference under such situation probably lies in the requirements for subsequent commercial registration and Health Insurance claims. With regard to the methodology of research in the pathways towards the proof of efficacy, what applies to treatment drug applies to health supplements.

5.3.5 *Fractionation Cocktails from Herbal Extracts*

One prominent difficulty in herbal medicine development lies in the need for QC. With a single chemical molecular drug, quality is maintained through chemical manufacture and evaluations. With botanical products, variations of the plant source are unavoidable. One might imagine optimistically that "good agricultural practice" (GAP) could ensure quality production. However, the limited scale of GAP practice and the variability of environments would not be able to satisfy the vast need for supplies (Leung and Cheng, 2008; Gao *et al.*, 2002; Huang *et al.*, 2002; Zhang *et al.*, 2010).

Research has started on ways to achieve better QC through platform productions like aqua-cultivation (Zhan and Lin, 2002).

Cheng at Yale has worked out a comprehensive testing platform for quality evaluation which satisfies regulatory needs, but would not ensure a quality supply. New attempts have started to better ensure quality supply of herbal products.

(i) *Combining fractionations with known marker chemicals instead of whole herb extracts*

Early trials have started to focus on the chemical markers of medicinal herbs in the attempt to ensure the quality of the herbs being used. Popular medicinal plants have known chemical markers which are used as hallmarks of genuineness. Known chemical maker can be identified from special fractionations. Hence, if the chemical markers are also responsible for the major biological activities, using the particular fractionations containing the markers, instead of the whole plant extract in the formulation of the herbal formulae would achieve much better quality assurance (QA).

In spite of the yet uncertainty that chemical and biological markers might not be identical, research and practice on this line is a logical attempt to achieve better QC of the herbs on both research and subsequently production levels (Zhou *et al.*, 1999; Shao *et al.*, 2004a, 2004b; Kang *et al.*, 2000; Bhuiyan and Sarkar, 1999).

(ii) *Cocultures*

Some medicinal plants like yeasts and fungi could be produced in special laboratories through fermentation or aqua-farming. If marker chemicals or specific fractionation products are added to the culture media, the cultivated mature plant may contain a quality store of the desired chemicals. This interesting research work has started (Bisset, 1994).

5.4 Difficulties Encountered in Research and Development of Chinese Medicine

Given the diversities of research possibilities related to Chinese herbal medicine, one might attain an impression that prosperous activities are ongoing. As a matter of fact, research activities have been limited to the drug discovery area motivated by phytochemists and pharmacologists. TCM practitioners are not keen on research because of their firm trust on old formulae. As new products of pharmaceuticals are in constant supply, clinicians in hospitals are already busy using the new drugs. They would not bother about possibilities and promises from traditional medicinal herbs.

This could be the background behind TM that urged the WHO to deliver the WHO Traditional Medicines Strategy in 2002 which focuses on four areas to be emphasised so that TM could play a better role in public health. The four areas are:

(a) Making national policy and regulations.
(b) Ensuring safety, efficacy and quality.
(c) Making traditional practice accessible to all.
(d) Offering training and facilitating communication between the traditional and modern streams.

The support on the four areas of concern has not been uniform in China and outside. Policies and regulations are plentiful, but the true integration between the traditional and modern streams is not maturing. Research activities to allow safety, efficacy and quality to be assured are yet to be desired.

5.5 Conclusions

With the many successes in the past of drug discovery from botanical origins, the popular use of proprietary herbal drug and with the rising popularity of health supplements, medicinal herbs should have a bright future for better and more innovative developments. The strong historical background and the rich collections of classical records on the clinical uses of herbs in Chinese medicine should be adequately encouraging strong commitments from both the academic and industrial sectors (Jaeschke *et al.*, 1989; Lai, 1998).

For the pharmaceutical industry, the never ending efforts on drug discovery exercises relying on small chemical molecules from herbs would continue. No other groups could afford the financial and human resources that are mandatorily required (Natasha, 2011).

For the smaller industries involved in the production of proprietary botanical preparations inherited from traditional herbal formulae, apart from maintaining the trust and confidence on the clinical value of the rich collections, they could bravely face the scientific challenges of the current era to upgrade the qualities and, more importantly, to support more evidence-based developments. The users of proprietary items deserve to have their personal selections basing on objective scientific evidences (Diplock, 1999; Clydesdale, 1997; Codex Alimentarius, 1997; AACE, 2003).

The academies tend to get contented with rich publications of scientific reports they produce concerning herb qualities, mechanisms of action and clinical effects. They may not realise that their academic endeavours should best be linked with market production so that people could enjoy their research findings.

Since the academics are not capable of capital mobilisations, they need to respond to the community need as well as the industries' requirements for expert services. In this vast field of health maintenance

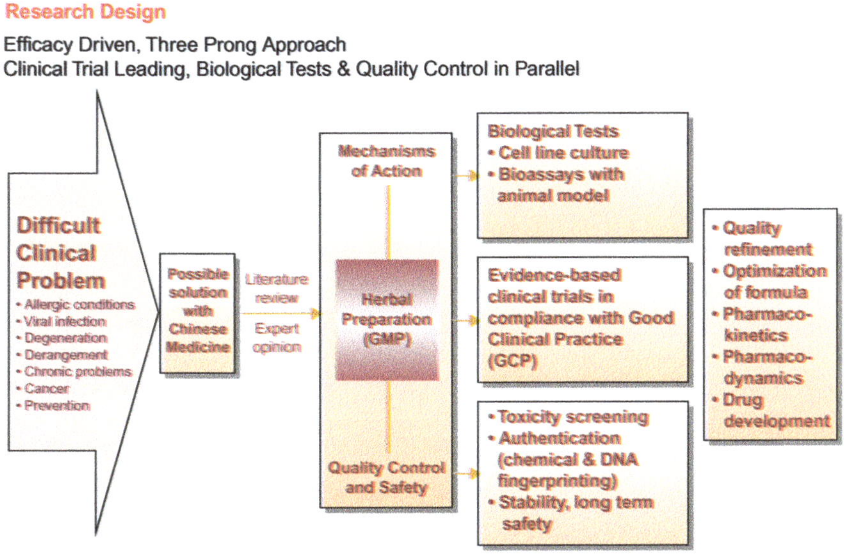

Figure 5.7. Research Approach for undertaking in the production of botanical items.

using medicinal herbs, the research platforms already established for drug discovery are suitable for the innovative development of better and evidence-based health supplements, starting with quality controls, exploring the mechanisms of action and eventually clinical evaluations. The comprehensive approach of research undertakings would result in the production of botanical items that people having special needs could safely rely on (Fig. 5.7).

With the ever increasing aging population the world over, age-related degenerations are as important as illnesses and endemics. Now that allopathic medicine based on single pathological targets is clearly not the only way to maintain health, TM and medicinal herbs have a lot to offer towards the maintenance of physiological harmony and the support against tissue and organ deteriorations. Medicinal herbs for longevity would find more and more practical applications (Sagar, 2001; Schipper *et al.*, 1995; Tagliaferri *et al.*, 2001; Wu *et al.*, 2005).

While functional food and nutritional support for health have gained general support for centuries, research with an evidence-based methodology similar to that of drug discovery is a new challenge. Perhaps, the health influence of specific botanical items which are capable of lowering disease risks is dependent on a gradual mechanism similar to that of metronomic chemotherapy, designed as slow, mild and gradual interventions, which, however, could still be put under objective evaluations (Kerbel and Kamen, 2004; Macek, 1984).

References

Aggett, P.J., Antoine, J.M., Asp, N.G. *et al.* (2005). Process for the assessment of scientific support for claims on foods (PASSCLAIM)–Consensus on Criteria. *Eur. J. Nutr.* **44**(1 Suppl), i5–i30.

American Association of clinical Endocrinologists (AACE) (2003). Medical guidelines for the clinical use of dietary supplements and nutraceuticals. *Endocrine practice* **9**(5), 417–470.

Beinfield, H. and Korngold, E. (1991). *Between Heaven and Earth: A Guide to Chinese Medicine.* Ballantine Books, New York.

Bisset, N.G. (1994). *Herbal Drugs and Phytopharmaceuticals.* CRC Press, Boca Raton.

Boik, J. (1996). *Cancer and Natural Medicine: A Textbook of Basic Science and Clinical Research.* Oregon Medical Press, Princeton.

Campion, E.W. (1993). Why unconventional medicine?" *N. Engl. J. Med.* **328**(4), 282–283.

Chan, Y.L., Woo, K.S., Leung, P.C. *et al.* (2006). Traditional Chinese medicine danshen and gegen combination formula improves atherogenic pathophysiology: an *in-vitro* and *ex-vivo* study. *J. HK. Coll. Cardiol.* **14**(2), 68.

Cheng, K.F. and Leung, P.C. (2011). Use of Chinese herbal medicine as an adjuvant for cancer treatment: a randomized controlled dose-finding clinical trial on lung cancer patients. *J. Cancer Ther.* **2**, 91–98.

Cheng, Y.C. (2003). Globalisation of Chinese medicine. In: *Comprehensive Guide to Chinese Medicine.* World Scientific Publishing Co. Pte. Ltd, Singapore.

Cheung, W.S.D., Koon, C.M., Ng, C.F. *et al.* (2012). The roots of *Salvia miltiorrhiza* (danshen) and *Pueraria lobata* (gegen) inhibit atherogenic events: A study of the combination effects of the 2-herb formula. *J. Ethnopharmacol.* **143**(3), 859–866.

Cheung, W.S.D., Koon, C.M., Wat, E. *et al.* (2013). A herbal formula containing roots of *Salvia miltiorrhiza* (danshen) and *Pueraria lobata* (gegen) inhibits inflammatory mediators in LPS-stimulated RAW 264.7 macrophages through inhibition of nuclear factor KB (NFkB) pathway. *J. Ethnopharmacol.* **145**, 776–783.

Clydesdale, F.M. (1997). A proposal for the establishment of scientific criteria for health claims for functioinal foods. *Nutr. Res.* **55**(12), 413–422.

Codex Alimentarius (1997). Codex guidelines for use of nutrition and health claims (CAC/GL 23-1997, Rev. 1–2004). Codex Alimentarius. WHO, Geneva.

Crutchley, R.D., Miller, J. and Garey, K.W. (2010). Crofelemer, a novel agent for treatment of secretory diarrhea. *Ann. Pharmacother.* **44**(5), 878–884.

Diplock, A.T. (Eds.) (1999). Scientific concepts of functional foods in Europe — consensus document. *Br. J. Nutr.* **81**(1), 1–27.

Eisenberg, D.M., Kessler, R.C., Foster, C. *et al.* (1993). Unconventional medicine in the United States. Prevalence, costs and patterns of use. *N. Engl. J. Med.* **328**(4), 246–252.

Endo, S., Nishida, T., Nishikawa, K. *et al.* (2006). Dai-kenchu-to, a Chinese herbal medicine, improves statsis of patients with total gastrectomy and jejunal pouch interposition. *Am. J. Surg.* **192**(1), 9–13.

Fair, W.R. (1999). The role of complementary medicine in urology. *J. Urol.* **162**, 411–420.

FDA approves first anti-diarrheal drug for HIV/AIDS patients (press release). (2012). US Food and Drug Administration, Silver Spring, MD. Available at: www.fda.gov/NewsEvents/Newsroom/PressAnnouncements/ucm333701.htm?source=govdelivery. Accessed Nov 30, 2013.

Feng, G.F., Tsu, L. (1972). *Tao Te Ching*. Vintage Books, New York.

Fiehn, O. (2002). Metabolomics — the link between genotypes and phenotypes. *Plant Mol. Biol.*, **48**(1–2), 155–171.

Fong, C.C., Wei, F., Chen, Y. *et al.* (2011). Danshen–Gegen decoction exerts proliferative effect on rat cardiac myoblasts H9c2 via MAPK and insulin pathways. *J. Ethnopharmacol.* **138**(1), 60–66.

Fu, W.K. (1985). *Traditional Chinese Medicine and Pharmacology*. Foreign Languages Press, Beijing.

Gao, W., Wei, J., Duan, H.Q. *et al.* (2002). Good Agriculture Practice (GAP) and sustainable resource utilization of Chinese materia medica. *J. Plant Biotechnol.* **4**(3), 103–107.

Goldbeck-Wood, S. and Dorozynski, A. (1996). Complementary medicine is booming worldwide. *BMJ*. **313**, 131.

Heyn, B. (1987). *Ayurvedic Medicine: The Gentle Strength of Indian Healing*. Thorsons Publishers, Wellingborough.

Hoizey, D. and Hoizey, M.J. (1988). *A History of Chinese Medicine*. Edinburgh University Press, Edinburgh.

Hood, L. (1998). Systems biology, new opportunities arising from genomics, proteomics and beyond. *Exp. Hematol.* **26**(8), 681–681.

Huang, L.Q., Cui, G.H., Chan, M.L. *et al.* (2002). Study on complex system of Chinese material medica GAP fulfilling the situation, problems, and prospects of Chinese material medica germplasm. *China Journal of Chinese Materia Medica* **27**, 481–483.

Huard, P. and Wong, M. (1968). *Chinese Medicine*. Weidenfeld and Nicolson, London.

Ichiko, F. (2011). Japan: Will the sun set on Kampo? *Nature* **480**, S96.

Ideker, T., Galitski, T. and Hood, L. (2001). A new approach to decoding life: systems biology. *Annu. Rev. Genomics Hum. Genet.* **2**, 343–372.

Itoh, T., Yamakawa, J., Mai, M. *et al.* (2002). The effect of the herbal medicine dai-kenchu-to on post-operative ileus. *J. Int. Med. Res.* **30**(4), 428–432.

Iwai N., Kume, Y. Kimura, O. *et al.* (2007). Effects of herbal medicine Dai-Kenchu-to on anorectal function in children with severe constipation. *Eur. J. Pediatr. Surg.* **17**(2), 115–118.

Jaeschke, R., Singer, J. and Guyatt, G.H. (1989). Measurement of health status. Ascertaining the minimal clinically important difference. *Control. Clin. Trials.* **10**(4), 407–415.

Jaggi, O.P. (1981). *History of Science, Technology and Medicine in India: Science in ancient India*. Atma Ram & Sons, Delhi.

Japanese Pharmacopoeia Fourteenth Edition (JP14), English version. (2002). Ministry of Health, Labour and Welfare, Government of Japan.

Kang, K., Kang, B., Lee, B. *et al.* (2000). Preventive effect of epicatechin and ginsenoside Rb(2) on the inhibition of gap junctional intercellular communication by TP and H2O2. *Cancer Lett.* **152**(1), 97–106.

Kaptchuk, T.J. and Eisenberg, D.M. (1998). The persuasive appeal of alternative medicine. *Ann. Intern. Med.* **129**(12), 1061–1065.

Kerbel, R.S. and Kamen, B.A. (2004). The anti-angiogenic basis of metronomic chemotherapy. *Nat. Rev. Cancer.* **4**, 423–436.

Kono, T., Kanematsu, T., Kitajima, M. (2009). Exodus of Kampo, traditional Japanese medicine, from the complementary and alternative medicines: is it time yet?" *Surgery* **146**(5), 837–840.

Kono, T., Koseki, T., Chiba, S. *et al.* (2008). Colonic vascular conductance increased by Daikenchuto via calcitonin gene-related peptide and receptor-activity modifying protein 1. *J. Surg. Res.* **150**(1), 78–84.

Koon, C.M., Woo, K.S., Leung, P.C. *et al.* (2011). Salviae Miltiorrhizae Radix and Puerariae Lobatae Radix herbal formula mediates anti-atherosclerosis by modulating key atherogenic events both in vascular smooth muscle cells and endothelial cells. *J. Ethnopharmacol.* **138**(1), 175–183.

Koon, C.M., Ko, C.H., Sun, X.X. *et al.* (2013). Gene expression profiling on the molecular action of danshen-gegen formula in a randomized placebo-controlled trial of postmenopausal women with hypercholesterolemia. *Evid. Based Complement. Alternat. Med.* **2013**, 703705.

Kuo, M.C., Weng, C.Y., Ha, C.L. *et al.* (2006). *Ganoderma lucidum* mycelia enhance inate immunity by activating NF-kappaB. *J. Ethnopharmacol.* **103**(2), 217–222.

Lai, S.L. (1998). *Clinical Trials of Traditional Chinese Materia Medica.* Guangdong People's Publishing House, China.

Lai, S.L. (2001). *Clinical Trials of Traditional Chinese Materia Medica.* Guangdong People's Publishing House, China

Lam, F.F.Y., Deng, S.Y., Ng, E.S.K. *et al.* (2010a). Mechanisms of the relaxant effect of a danshen and gegen formulation on rat isolated cerebral basilar artery. *J. Ethnopharmacol.* **132**(1), 186–192.

Lam, W., Bussom, S., Guan, F. *et al.* (2010b). The four-herb Chinese medicine PHY906 reduces chemotherapy-induced gastrointestinal toxicity. *Sci. Transl. Med.*, **2**(45), 45ra59.

Law, W., Bussom, S. and Cheng, Y.C. (2009). Effect of hypoxia on the expression of phosphoglycerate kinase and antitumor activity of troxacitabine and gemcitabine in non-small cell lung carcinoma. *Mol. Cancer Biol.* **8**(2), 415–423.

Leung, P.C. (2001). Editorial-seminar series on evidence-based alternative medicine. *Hong Kong Med. J.* 7(4), 332–334.

Leung P.C. (2008). *Developing Hong Kong into a Chinese Medicine International Platform — A careful study.* Central Policy Unit Publication, the Government of Hong Kong Special Administrative Region.

Leung, P.C and Cheng, K.F. (2008). Good Agricultural Practice (GAP) –does it ensure a perfect supply of medicinal herbs for research and drug development? *International Journal of Applied Research in Natural Products* **1**(2), 1–8.

Leung, P.C., Chook, P., Kwong, S.K. *et al.* (2010). Adjunctive danshen and Gegen Therapy Improves Atherogenic Process: A Final Report of Double-blind Placebo Control Trial in High Risk Hypertension. In: *The 23rd Scientific meeting of the International Society of Hypertension-WHL anc CHL Joint Symposium*, Vancouver, BC.

Leung, P.C., Koon, C.M., Lau, C.B.S. *et al.* (2013). Ten years' research on a cardiovascular tonic: a comprehensive approach — from quality control and mechanisms of action to clinical trial. *Evid. Based Complement. Alternat. Med.* **2013**, 319703.

Li, J., Zhang, Z., Rosenzweig, J. *et al.* (2002). Proteomics and bioinformatics approaches for identification of serum biomarkers to detect breast cancer. *Clin. Chem.* **48**(8), 1296–1304.

Liang, W., Teong, I.W.J., Koon, C.M. *et al.* (2012). Inhibitory effects of salviae miltiorrhizae radix (danshen) and puerariae lobatae radix (gegen) in carbachol-induced rat detrusor smooth muscle contractility. *Int. J. Physiol. Pathophysiol. Pharmacol.* **4**(1), 36–44.

Liu, S.H. and Cheng, Y.C. (2012). Old formula, new Rx: The journal of PHY906 as cancer adjuvant therapy. *J. Ethnopharmacol.* **140**, 614–623.

Luo, G.A. and Wang, Y.M. (1997). Research methods and theory on effective component groups of TCM formulae. *Chinese Traditional Patent Medicine* **8**, 44–45.

Luo, G.A. and Wang, Y.M. (1999). The study on relationship between chemical substance basis and pharmacological effect of TCM formulae. *World Science and Technology: Modernization of Traditional Chinese Medicine and Materia Medica* **1**, 11–15.

Luo, G.A., Wang, Y.M., Liang, Q.L. *et al.* (2012). *Systems Biology for Traditional Chinese Medicine.* John Wiley & Sons Inc., New Jersey.

Macek, C. (1984). East meets West to balance immunologic yin and yang. *JAMA* **251**(4), 433–441.

Manabe, N., Camilleri, M., Rao, A., *et al.* (2010). Effect of daikenchuto (TU-100) on gastrointestinal and colonic transit in humans. *Am. J. Physiol. Gastrointest. Liver Physiol.* **298**(6), G970–975.

Mangel, A.W. and Chaturvedi, P. (2008). Evaluation of crofelemer in the treatment of diarrhea-predominant irritable bowel syndrome patients. *Digestion* **78**(4), 180–186.

McGrew, R. (1985). *Encyclopedia of Medical History.* Mcgraw-Hill.

Nagano, T., Itoh, H. and Takeyama, M. (1999). Effect of *Dai-kenchu-to* on levels 3 brain-gut peptides (motilin, gastrin and somatostatin) in human plasma. *Biol. Pharm. Bull.* **22**(10), 1131–1133.

Natasha, G. (2011). Reglations: Herbal medicine rule book. *Nature* **480**, S98–S99.

Ng, C.F., Koon, C.M., Cheung, W.S.D., *et al.* (2011). The Anti-hypertensive effect of danshen (*Salvia miltiorrhiza*) and gegen (*Pueraria lobata*) formula in rats and its underlying mechanisms of vasorelaxation. *J. Ethnopharmacol.* **137**, 1366–1372.

Nicholson, J.K., Lindon, J.C. and Holmes, E. (1999). Metabonomics: understanding the metabolic responses of living systems to pathophysiological stimuli via multivariate statistical analysis of biological NMR spectroscopic data. *Xenobiotica* **29**(11), 1181–1189.

Quella, S.K., Loprinzi, C.L., Barton, D.L., *et al.* (2000). Evaluation of soy phytoestrogens for the treatment of hot flashes in breast cancer survivors: A north central cancer treatment group trial. *J. Clin. Oncol.* **18**(5), 1068–1074.

Rockwell, S., Grove, T.A., Liu, Y.F., *et al.* (2013). Preclinical studies of the Chinese medicine formulation PHY906 as a potential adjunct to radiation therapy. *Int. J. Radiat. Biol.* **89**(1), 16–25.

Sagar, S.M. (2001). *Restored Harmony: An Evidence-based Approach For Integrating Traditional Chinese Medicine into Complementary Cancer Care.* Dreaming DragonFly Communications, Canada, Ontario.

Schepetkin, I.A. and Quinn, M.T. (2006). Botanical polysaccharides: Macrophage immunomodulation and therapeutic potential. *Int. Immunopharmacol.* **6**, 317–333.

Schipper, H., Goh, C.R. and Wang, T.L. (1995). Shifting the cancer paradigm: Must we kill to cure?" *J. Clin. Oncol.* **13**, 801–807.

Shao, B.M., Dai, H., Xu, W., *et al.* (2004a). Immune receptors for polysaccharides from *Ganoderma lucidum. Biochem. Biophys. Res. Commun.* **323**(1), 133–141.

Shao, B.M., Xu, W., Dai, H. *et al.* (2004b). A Study on the immune receptors for polysaccharides from the roots of *Astragalus membranceus*, a Chinese medicinal herb. *Biochem. Biophys. Res. Commun.* **320**(4), 1103–1111.

Shibata, C., Sasaki, I., Naito, H., *et al.* (1999). The herbal medicine *Dai-Kenchu-to* stimulates upper gut motility through cholinergic and 5-hydroxytryptamine 3 receptors in conscious dogs. *Surgery* **126**(5), 918–924.

Stephens, F.O. (1999). The rising incidence of breast cancer in women and prostate cancer in men. Dietary influence: A possible preventive role for nature's sex hormone modifiers-the phytoestrogens. *Oncol. Rep.* **6**(4), 865–870.

Tagliaferri, M., Cohen, I. and Tripathy, D. (2001). Complementary and alternative medicine in early-stage breast cancer. *Semin. Oncol.* **28**(1), 121–134.

Taira, Z., Yabe, K., Hamaguchi, Y., *et al.* (2004). Effects of *Sho-saiko-to* extract and its components, Baicalin, baicalein, glycyrrhizin and glycyrrhetic acid, on pharmacokinetic behavior of salicylamide in carbon tetrachloride intoxicated rats. *Food Chem. Toxicol.* **42**(5), 803–807.

Takakusu, J. (1956). Observation of Medicine in India and China. In: *History of Science in India.* Editorial Enterprises, New Delhi.

Tam, W.Y., Chook, P., Qiao, M., *et al.* (2009). The efficacy and tolerability of adjunctive alternative herbal medicine (*Salvia miltiorrhiza* and *Pueraria lobata*) on vascular function and structure in coronary patients. *J. Altern. Complement. Med.* **15**(4), 415–421.

Tang, W. and Eisenberg, G. (1992). *Chinese Drugs of Plant Origin: Chemistry, Pharmacology and Use in Traditional and Modern Medicine.* Springer-Verlag, New York.

Tatti, S., Swinehart, J.M., Thielert, C., *et al.* (2008). Sinecatechins, a defined green tea extract, in the treatment of external anogenital warts: a randomized controlled trial. *Obstet. Gynecol.* **111**(6), 1371–1379.

Terauchi, M., Hiramitsu, S., Akiyoshi, M., *et al.* (2011). Effects of three Kampo formulae: Tokishakuyakusan(TJ-23), Kamishoyosan(TJ-24) and Keishibukuryoan(TJ-25) on Japanese peri-and postmenopausal women with sleep disturbance. *Arch. Gynecol. Obstet.* **284**(4), 913–921.

Traditional Medicine, Essential Drugs and Medicines Policy (EDM). (2002). *WHO Traditional Medicine Strategy 2002–2005.* WHO, Geneva.

Tradtrantip, L., Namkung, W. and Verkman, A.S. (2010). Crofelemer, an antisecretory antidiarrheal proanthocyanidin oligomer extracted from *Croton lechleri*, targets two distinct intestinal chloride channels. *Mol. Pharmacol.* **77**(1), 69–78.

Tu, Y.Y. (2011). The discovery of artemisinin (*qinghaosu*) and gifts from Chinese Medicine. *Nat.Med.* **17**, 1217–1220.

Wang, E., Busson, S., Chen, J., *et al.* (2011). Interaction of a traditional Chinese Medicine (PHY906) and CPT-11 on the inflammatory process in the tumor microenvironment. *BMC med Genomics* **4**, 38.

Watanabe, K. (2007). Kampo Treatment for Cancer. *Asia Pac. Biotech.* **11**(17), 1186–1190.

Watanabe, S., Imanishi, J., Satoh, M. and Ozasa, K. (2001). Unique place of Kampo (Japanese traditional medicine) in complementary and alternative medicine: A survey of doctors belonging to the regional medical association in Japan. *Tohoku J. Exp. Med.* **194**(1), 55–63.

Watanabe, K., Matsuura, K., Gao, P.F., *et al.* (2011). Traditional Japanese Kampo Medicine: Clinical Research between Modernity and Traditional Medicine — The State of Research and Methodological Suggestions for the Future. *Evid. Based Complement. Alternat. Med.* **2011**, 51384.

WHO. (2000). Promoting the Role of Traditional medicine in Health Systems: A Strategy for the African Region. Fiftieth Session of the WHO Regional Committee.

Wong, C.K., Leung, K.N., Fung, K.P., *et al.* (1994). Immunomodulatory and antitumour polysaccharides from medicinal plants. *J. Int. Med. Res.* **22**(6), 299–312.

Wong, C.K., Bao, Y.X., Wong, E.L., *et al.* (2005). Immunomodulatory activities of yunzhi and danshen in post-treatment breast cancer patients. *Am. J. Chin. Med.* **33**(3), 381–395.

Wong, L.Y., Leung, P.C., Tang, J. L., *et al.* (2010). Use of dietary supplements by breast cancer patients undergoing conventional cancer treatment. *Patient Prefer. Adher.* **4**, 407–414.

Woo, K.S., Yip, T.W.C., Chook, P., *et al.* (2013). Cardiovascular Protective Effects of Adjunctive Alternative Medicine (*Salvia miltiorrhiza* and *Pueraria lobata*) in High-Risk Hypertension. *Evid. Based Complement. Alternat. Med.* **2013**, 132912.

Wood, M.J., Hyman, N.H. and Mawe, G.M. (2010). The effects of Daikenchuto (DKT) on Propulsive Motility in the colon. *J. Surg. Res.* **164**(1), 84–90.

Wu, T., Munro, A.J., Guanjian, L., *et al.* (2005). Chinese medical herbs for chemotherapy side effects in colorectal cancer patients. *Cochrane Database Syst. Rev.* **25**(1), CD004540.

Yang, C.S. and Wang, Z.Y. (1993). Tea and cancer. *J. Natl. Cancer Inst.* **85**(13), 1038–1049.

Yue, G.G.L., Lee, J.K.M., Cheng, L., *et al.* (2012). Reversal of P-glycoprotein-mediated multidrug resistance in human hepatoma cells by hedyotiscone A, a compound isolated from *Hedyotis corymbosa. Xenobiotica* **42**(6), 562–570.

Yue, G.G.L., Fan, J.T., Lee, J. K. M., *et al.* (2011). Cyclopeptide RA-V inhibits angiogenesis by down-regulating ERK1/2 phosphorylation in HUVEC and HMEC-1 endothelial cells. *Br. J. Pharmacol.* **164**(7), SI1883–1898.

Yun, T.K. and Choi, S.Y. (1998). Non-organ specific cancer prevention of ginseng: A prospective study in Korea. *Int. J. Epidemiol.* **27**(3), 359–364.

Zhan, N.P. and Lin, R.C. (2002). The establishment of SOP for different Chinese Materia Medica in China. *Res. Inform. Trad. Chin. Med.* **3**(3), 15–17.

Zhang, B.G., Yong, P., Zhang, Z., *et al.* (2010). GAP Production of TCM herbs in China. *Planta Med.* **76**(17), 1948–1955.

Zhang, J.F., He, M.L., Dong, Q. *et al.* (2011). Aqueous Extracts of *Fructus ligustri lucidi* enhance the sensitivity of human colorectal carcinoma DLD-1 cells to doxorubicin-induced apoptosis via tbx3 suppression. *Integr. Cancer. Ther.* **10**(1), 85–91.

Zhou, J.R., Gugger, E.T., Tanaka, T., *et al.* (1999). Soybean phytochemicals inhibit the growth of transplantable human prostate carcinoma and tumor angiogenesis in mice. *J. Nutr.* **129**(9), 1628–1935.

Zhou, L.M., Wang, S., Zhang, Z., *et al.* (2012). Pharmacokinetic and pharmacodynamic interaction of danshen–gegen extract with warfarin and aspirin. *J. Ethnopharmacol.* **143**(2), 648–655.

Chapter 6

Evidence-Based Validation of Indian Traditional Medicine: Way Forward*

Pulok K Mukherjee, Ranjit K Harwansh, Shiv Bahadur, Subhadip Banerjee and Amit Kar

Abstract

Evidence-based validation of the ethno-pharmacological claims on traditional medicine (TM) is the need of the day for its globalisation and reinforcement. Combining the unique features of identifying biomarkers that are highly conserved across species, this can offer an innovative approach to biomarker-driven drug discovery and development. TMs are an integral component of alternative health care systems. India has a rich wealth of TMs and the potential to accept the challenge to meet the global demand for them. Ayurveda, Yoga, Unani, Siddha and Homeopathy (AYUSH) medicine are the major healthcare systems in Indian TM. The plant species mentioned in the ancient texts of these systems may be explored with the modern scientific approaches for better leads in the healthcare. TM is the best source of chemical diversity for finding new drugs and leads. Authentication and scientific validation of medicinal plant is a fundamental requirement of industry and other organisations dealing with herbal drugs. Quality control (QC) of

* First published in World Journal of Traditional Chinese Medicine [*World J. Tradit. Chin. Med.* 2016, 2(1): 48–61]. DOI:10.15806/j.issn.2311-8571.2015.0018.

botanicals, validated processes of manufacturing, customer awareness and post-marketing surveillance are the key points, which would ensure the quality, safety and efficacy of TM. For globalisation of TM, there is a need for harmonisation with respect to its chemical and metabolite profiling, standardisation, QC, scientific validation, documentation and regulatory aspects of TM. Therefore, utmost attention is necessary for the promotion and development of TM through global collaboration and coordination by national and international programme.

Keywords: Indian Traditional Medicine; AYUSH; Ayurveda; Chemical Profiling; Plant Metabolomics.

6.1 Introduction

Traditional medicine (TM) has a long history of cultural heritage and ethnic practices. TM has been defined as skills and a practice based on the theories, believes and experiences indigenous to different cultures and maintenance of healthcare as well as in the prevention, diagnosis and treatment of physical and mental illnesses (Mukherjee *et al.*, 2012). Some evidences of efficacy, safety and quality, if they exist, for herbal medicines, are considered to be anecdotal or empirical at best and rarely it is subjected to the rigorous prospective randomised controlled trial. Until 1899, when Bayer introduced aspirin, traditional and ethno medicine was the basis of healthcare for humankind. Through a slow process of clinical trial and error, each culture developed a local, natural resource-based tradition of healing. These systems of TM, today, provide the basis of drug supply for an estimated 4.6 billion people worldwide (Cordell and Colvard, 2012).

All patients have the right to expect that a medicine will "work", i.e. it will be safe, effective and consistent. Ethically, it should not matter whether the medicine is an approved prescription product, over-the-counter medication, dietary supplement, phyto-pharmaceutical, or TM when human health is at stake. To diminish that right is to diminish the value of one human life over another. Global implementation of an evidence-based regulatory foundation for TMs and dietary supplements is essential to ensure healthcare for all (Mukherjee, 2001). Scientific validation and quality control (QC) of TMs are critical and essential aspects to ensure therapeutic efficacy, safety and rationalisation of their use in healthcare. Quality assurance (QA) is the thrust area for traditional formulations in Indian TM like *churnas* (herb powder), *bhasmas* (calcined metallic ashes), *Kwath* (liquid orals) and *Lehas* (oral supplements). Chromatographic finger printing and marker compound analysis are getting momentum for the standardisation of traditional medicinal formulations. This technique helps not only in establishing the correct botanical identity but also helps in regulating the chemical profile of the herbs (Mukherjee *et al.*, 2011). TMs have been regarded as stronghold in drug discovery and drug development as they offer unmatched chemical diversity with structural complexity and novel biological interactions. Searching for the TMs in untapped source can lead us to new horizons where we can find novel, potent and selective lead compounds. Such leveraging innovations in the development of TM products (TMPs) suggested an immense growth potential in future for their validation. The European Medicines Agency (EMA) defines chemical markers as chemically defined constituents or groups of constituents of herbal medicinal product, which are of interest for QC purposes in spite of whether or not they possess any therapeutic activity (Li *et al.*, 2008).

Wisdom and compassion, global collaboration and leadership are essential to change the contemporary paradigms and develop new strategies for the promotion of TMs. From the history on discovery and development of drugs, it is understood that with adequate support, an important health outcome of the evidence-based approach to the study of TMs has developed several safe and effective medicines (Afaq and Mukhtar, 2006). The rich secondary metabolite resources of medicinal plants are widely accepted for their unique chemical and biological features. They are gaining global acceptance because they offer natural ways of treatment and promote healthcare. Scientists around the world are emphasising on medicinal plants as alternative medicine and their commercial potential in healthcare (Mukherjee and Wahile, 2006).

6.2 Indian System of Medicine (ISM)

India has an ancient heritage of traditional system of medicine. Indian Materia-Medica provides a huge knowledge base on folklore practices of traditionally inspired medicine. Indian TM is based on Ayurveda, Yoga, Unani, Siddha and Homeopathy (AYUSH), with the emerging interest of the world in adopting and studying traditional systems, and in exploiting their potential from different healthcare perspectives, the Ministry of

AYUSH, Government of India has initiated several attempts to explore the possibility of evaluating TMs for their therapeutic potential as originally practised, as well as to generate data to put them in national healthcare programs. The Ministry of AYUSH regulates education, practice and encourages research in these systems. The National Medicinal Plant Board (NMPB) deals with conservation, cultivation, post-harvest technology and related issues on medicinal plants (Mukherjee *et al.*, 2010b). The detailed profile of Ministry of AYUSH, Government of India is given in Table 6.1.

Table 6.1. Various organisations of Ministry of AYUSH, Government of India for exploration and development of TM.

Organisations	Particulars
Research councils	♆ Central Council for Research in Ayurvedic Sciences (CCRAS), New Delhi ♆ Central Council for Research in Siddha (CCRS), Tamil Nadu ♆ Central Council for Research in Unani Medicines (CCRUM), New Delhi ♆ Central Council for Research in Homoeopathy (CCRH), New Delhi ♆ Central Council for Research in Yoga & Naturopathy (CCRYN), New Delhi
Board	❖ National Medicinal Plant Board (NMPB), New Delhi
Educational institutions	⚡ National Institute of Ayurveda (NIA), Jaipur ⚡ National Institute of Naturopathy (NIN), Pune ⚡ National Institute of Unani Medicine (NIUM), Bangalore ⚡ National Institute of Siddha (NIS), Chennai ⚡ National Institute of Homoeopathy (NIH), Kolkata ⚡ Institute of Post Graduate Teaching & Research in Ayurveda (IPGTRA), Jamnagar, Gujarat ⚡ Rashtriya Ayurveda Vidyapeeth (RAV), New Delhi ⚡ Morarji Desai National Institute of Yoga (MDNIY), New Delhi
Statutory organisations	☼ The Central Council of Indian Medicine (CCIM), New Delhi ☼ The Central Council for Homoeopathy (CCH), New Delhi
Manufacturing unit	❖ Indian Medicine Pharmaceutical Corporation Ltd. (IMPCL), Almora, Uttarakhand
Laboratories	★ Pharmacopoeial Laboratory for Indian Medicine (PLIM), Ghaziabad, UP ★ Homoeopathic Pharmacopoeia Laboratory (HPL), Ghaziabad, UP

India has approximately 47,000 plant species and about 15,000 medicinal plants, among them 7,000 plants used in Ayurveda, 700 in Unani medicine, 600 in Siddha medicine. The 65% population in rural India is using Ayurvedic medicines. Traditionally, 2,000 species in Ayurveda, Siddha and Unani (ASU) medicine are used by classical traditions. Traditional village practitioners are practising 4,500–5,000 species. Tribal and other traditional communities use 8,000 plant species. The details of herbs used the in Indian system of medicine have been described in Fig. 6.1. Medicinal Plants Division of the Indian Council of Medical Research (ICMR) has brought out 13 volumes in a series of publications entitled "Reviews on Indian Medicinal Plants" consolidating multidisciplinary scientific published research work on 3,679 Indian medicinal plant species with 56,964 citations on various aspects including pharmacognostic, ethnobotanicals, Ayurvedic, phytochemical, pharmacology and toxicology.

AYUSH are the official Indian traditional systems of medicine. The Department of Indian Systems of Medicines and Homoeopathy (ISM & H) was established in March, 1995 as a separate department in the Indian Ministry of Health and Family Welfare and re-named as Department of (AYUSH) in November 2003 with a view to providing focused attention to development of Education and Research in AYUSH. The Department has been elevated to an independent ministry w.e.f. 09.November.2014. The

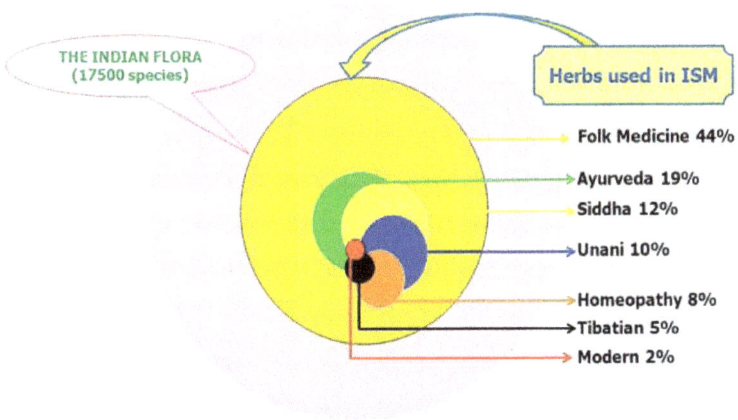

Figure 6.1. TM used in Indian system of medicine.

ministry continues to lay emphasis on upgradation of AYUSH educational standards, QC and standardisation of drugs, improving the availability of medicinal plant material, research and development and awareness generation about the efficacy of the products of the systems (AYUSH, 2015).

Under the Ministry of AYUSH, there are five research councils, one board, eight educational institutions, two statutory organisations, one drug manufacturing unit, two laboratories, and 11 national institutes established at national level for promoting current research, clinical practices and related aspects (Chatterjee, 2012). Various sectors of Ministry of AYUSH, Government of India for promotion and development of TM are given in Table 6.1.

6.2.1 *Ayurveda*

Ayurveda, the "Science of life", is accepted as one of the oldest treatises on medical systems came into existence in about 900 B.C. According to Indian Hindu mythology, there are four *Vedas* written by the Aryans — *Rig veda, Shama veda, Yajur veda,* and *Atharva veda.* Among these, *Rig veda,* the oldest, was written after 1500 B.C. The Ayurveda is said to be an *Upaveda* (part) of Atharva veda, whereas the *Charak Samhita* (1900 B.C.) is the first recorded treatise fully devoted to the concepts of practice of Ayurveda (Anonymous, 2001). According to Ayurveda, a human being is a replica of nature and everything, which affects the human body and influences the macrocosm. Along with these *Panchamahabhutas,* the functional aspect like movement, transformation and growth is governed by three biological humours, *viz. vata* (space and air), *pitta* (fire and water) and *kapha* (water and earth), respectively. This phenomenon may be attributed to the philosophy in Ayurveda known as *Ashtanga Ayurveda.* In Ayurveda, major disciplines are *Ayurveda Siddhanta* (fundamental principles of Ayurveda), *Ayurveda Samhita* (dealing with Ayurvedic classics), *Sharira Rachna* (anatomy), *Sharira Kriya* (physiology), *Dravya Guna Vigyan* (Materia Medica and pharmacology), *Rasa Shastra* (metal and minerals processing), *Bhaishajya Kalpana* (pharmaceuticals), *Kaumarabhritya* (paediatrics), *Prasuti Tantra* (obstetrics and gynaecology), *Swasthavritta* (social and preventive medicine), *Kayachikitsa* (internal medicines), *Roga Nidana* (etiopathology), *Shalya Tantra* (surgery), *Shalkya Tantra* (eye and ENT),

Manasa Roga (psychiatry), *Agada Tantra* (toxicology and forensic medicine), *Sangaharana* (anaesthesia) and *Panchakarma* (cleansing for rejuvenation therapy). Ayurveda is widely respected for its uniqueness and global acceptance as it offers natural ways to treat diseases and promote health (Mukherjee *et al.*, 2012; Debnath *et al.*, 2015). The major discipline in Ayurveda has been explained in Fig. 6.2.

Ayurveda is heath care in continuity since Indus Valley Civilisation (2300–1750 B.C.). We must consider human being as a whole with body, mind and soul to be healthy; healthy life is ensured by the harmony of these three entities. In life, we must have satisfaction of mind and tranquillity of spirit. In Ayurveda, all recipes have been given; one has to find out the right things in the right directions. Ayurveda considers individual as a whole, the object of treatment, and not merely a particular expression of

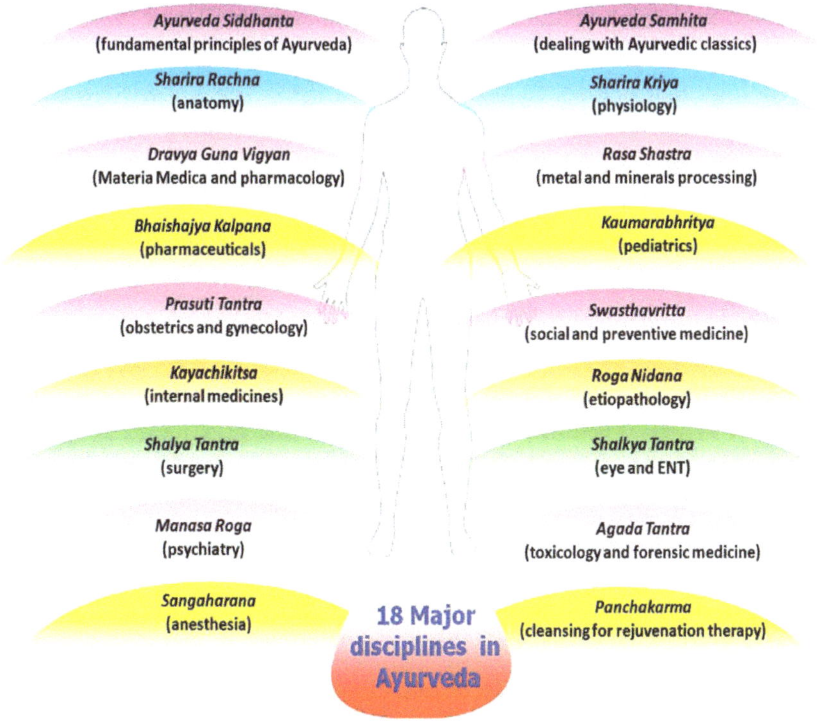

Figure 6.2. Major disciplines in Ayurveda.

that system. In order to understand Ayurveda, we need scientific thinking which in turn will answer various health care issues (Debnath *et al.*, 2015).

The backbone of Ayurveda can be traced to the beginning of cosmic creation. In the earth, everything is composed of matter (substance), and as per the Ayurveda, all matter consists of five basic elements (*Panchamahabhutas*): the first element is space (*Akasha*), and the remaining four elements are air (*vayu*), water (*jala*), fire (*agni*) and earth (*prithivi*) which exist within the space. Both the systems, human (microcosm) and universe (macrocosm), are linked permanently, since both are built from the same elements. Thus, humans are miniatures of the universe, a replica of nature, and everything that affects human beings also influences the macrocosm. Hence, the evolution of life and the creation of the universe can be concerned with Ayurveda. Along with these *Panchamahabhutas*, functional aspects like movement, transformation, and growth are governed by three biological humours, *viz. Vata* (space and air), *pitta* (fire and water) and *kapha* (water and earth), respectively. These three bodily humours usually known as *Tridhatus* regulate every physiological and psychological processes in the living organism. The knowledge base of Ayurveda includes Ayurvedic medicine, Ayurvedic principles, therapeutic modalities *Panchakarma*, and preventive aspect through *Rasayana* and veterinary use (Debnath *et al.*, 2015).

6.2.2 *Siddha*

The Siddha is one of the ancient systems of traditional Indian medicine. The term 'Siddha' means achievement and the "Siddhars" were saintly figures who achieved results in medicine through the practices. The system is believed to be developed by 18 "Siddhars", who glorified human being as the highest form of birth and believed that preserving the human body is essential to achieve the eternal bliss. The principles and concepts of this system are closely similar to those of Ayurveda, with specialisation in iatrochemistry. As in Ayurveda, This system also considers the human body as a conglomeration of three humours, seven basic tissues and the waste products. The equilibrium of humours is considered as health and its disturbance or imbalance leads to disease or sickness. The system describes 96 chief constituents of a human being, which include physical, physiological, moral and intellectual components. When there is any change or disturbance in functioning of these principals, body as a system deviates towards the cause of disease. The diagnostic methodology in the Siddha system is eight-fold, including examination of pulse, tongue, complexion, speech, palpatory findings, and so forth. Perception has a great role in this venture; this can be achieved by sensory organs, by mind, by yoga, by pain and pleasure. The Siddha system is a psychosomatic system, where attention is given to minerals and metals along with plant constituents (Mukherjee and Wahile, 2006).

6.2.3 *Unani*

The Unani system of medicine owes its origin in Greece. In India, Arabs introduced the Unani system of medicine, which was developed and blended with the Indian culture under the Mughal Emperors. The Greek philosopher-physician Hippocrates (460–377 B.C.), Greek and Arab scholars like Galen (131–212 A.D.), Raazes (850–0925 A.D.) and Avicenna (980–1037 A.D.) enriched this system considerably. Unani considers the human body to be made up of seven components. *Arkan* — elements, *Mizaj* — temperaments, *Aklath* — humours, *Anza* — organs, *Arawh* — spirits, *Quo* — faculties and *Afal* — functions, each of which has a close relationship with the state of health of an individual. A physician takes into account all these factors before diagnosing and prescribing treatment. In Unani medicine, single drugs or their combinations are preferred over compound formulations. The naturally occurring drugs used in this system are symbolic of life and are generally free from side effects. Such drugs, which are toxic in crude form, are processed and purified in many ways before use (Mukherjee and Wahile, 2006).

In Unani system of medicines, the diseases are considered as a natural process, and their symptoms are the reaction of the body. Therefore, the chief function of the physician is to aid the natural forces of the body. This system believes that every person has a unique humour constitution, which represents his healthy state. Hippocrates was the first physician to introduce the method of taking medical histories, which gave rise to the development of "humoral theory" and presumed the presence of several humours such as *Dam* (blood) *Balgham* (phlegm), *Safra* (yellow bile) and

Sauda (black bile) in the body. The Unani system believes that every person has a unique humoral constitution that represents its healthy state. There is power of self-preservation or adjustment called the "vis medicatrix natuare" or the vis defenae mechanism, which strives to restore disturbances within the limit prescribed by the constitution of an individual and imbalance in the humour systems lead to several diseases (Mukherjee and Wahile, 2006).

6.2.4 *Homoeopathy*

Homoeopathy as it is practised today was evolved by the German physician, Dr. Samuel Hahnemann (1755–1843). The word "Homoeopathy" is derived from two Greek words, *Homois* meaning similar and *Pathos* meaning suffering. Homoeopathy simply means treating diseases with remedies, which are capable of producing symptoms similar to the disease when taken by healthy people. Homoeopathy is being practised since ≥150 years in India. It has blended so well into the roots and traditions of the country that it has been recognised as one of the system of medicine and plays an essential role in boosting human healthcare largely (Mukherjee and Wahile, 2006).

6.3 Leveraging Approaches for Validation of Traditional Medicine

The practices and public interest in natural therapies and TM have increased dramatically. This has increased international trade in herbal medicine and attracted number of pharmaceutical companies. A few years ago, only small companies had interest in the marketing of TM, now multinational companies have started showing interest in commercialising herbal drugs (Heyman and Meyer, 2012).

In traditional systems of medicine, the medicinal plants play a major role and constitute their backbone. Indian Materia-Medica includes about 2,000 drugs of natural origin almost all of which are derived from different traditional systems and folklore practices (Narayana *et al.*, 1998). According to WHO reports, the population in developing countries like India (70%), Rwanda (70%), Uganda (60%), Tanzania (60%), Benin (80%) and Ethiopia

(90%) use traditional and alternative medicines for health care. In developed countries like Belgium (31%), USA (42%), Australia (48%), France (49%), Canada (70%), a significant percentage of the population has used traditional and alternative remedies for healthcare (WHO, 2004). The global market of trade related to medicinal plants is estimated around US $60 billion per year and is growing at the rate of 7% annually with varying shares of developed and developing countries (Raskin *et al.*, 2002).

Discovery of new drugs is facing serious challenges due to reduction in the number of new drug approvals coupled with excessive increasing cost. Combinatorial chemistry provided new expectation of higher achievement rates of new chemical entities (NCEs) but this scientific development has failed to improve the success rate in novel drug discovery. This scenario has prompted researchers to come out with a novel approach of integrated drug discovery. The starting point for plant-based new drug discovery should be identification of the right candidate plants by applying traditional documented use, tribal non-documented use, and exhaustive literature search. Bioassay-guided fractionation of the identified plant may lead to standardised extract or isolated bioactive compound as the new drug. This integrated approach could enhance success rate in drug discovery (Katiyar *et al.*, 2012). The development of TM requires the convergence of modern techniques and integrated approaches related to their evidence based research in various fields of science through national and international coordination (Mukherjee *et al.*, 2014a). The integrated strategies of drug development from TM have been enumerated in Fig. 6.3.

6.4 Approaches for Research and Development in Traditional Medicine

Around 25,000 effective plant-based formulations are used as folk medicine in different rural communities of India (Nema *et al.*, 2011) and about 95% of medicinal plants are obtained from wild sources, among them only 150 species are used commercially. Approximately, 5–15% of the total 250,000 species have been validated scientifically. The annual turnover of the Indian herbal medicinal industry is about Rs. 2,300 crore as against the pharmaceutical industry's turnover of Rs. 14,500 crores with a growth rate of 15%. There are over 1.5 million traditional practitioners and approximately 7,000

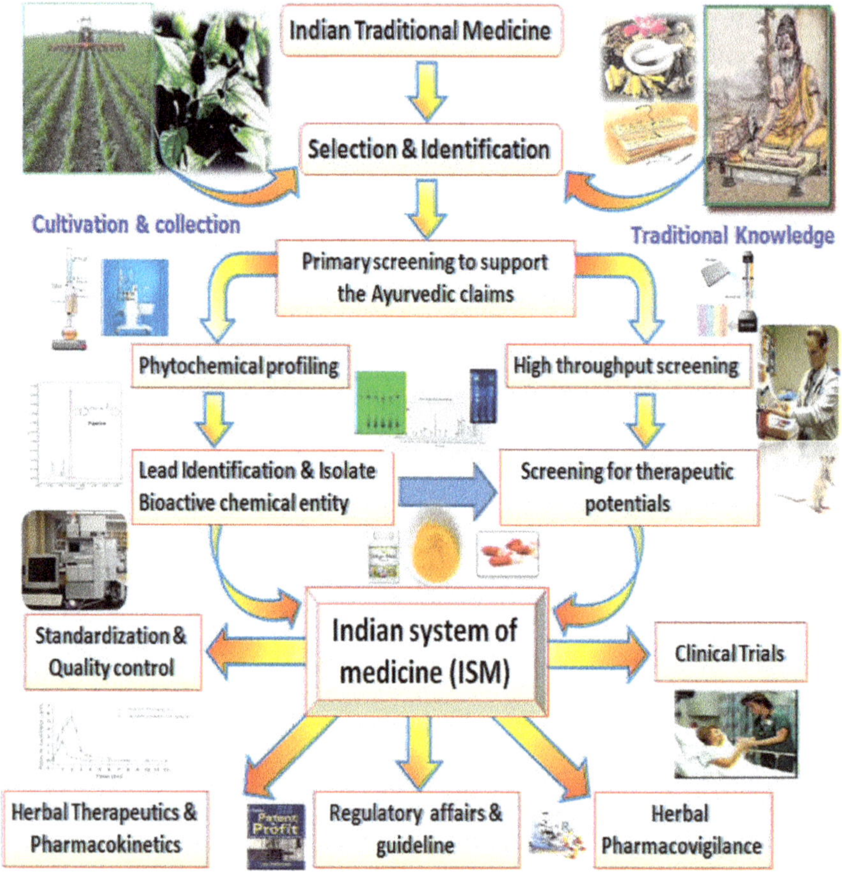

Figure 6.3. Leveraging approaches for the development of TM.

medicinal drug-manufacturing units, which are using medicinal plants for prevention and treatment of different ailments (Sen *et al.*, 2011).

Major thrust areas of research in TM includes: (i) phytochemical and pharmacological screening, (ii) chemo-profiling, (iii) DNA-bar coding, (iv) phyto-informatics, (v) metabolomic study, (vi) phyto-equivalence, (vii) reverse pharmacology, (viii) high-throughput screening, (ix) safety evaluation, (x) value added drug delivery system; (xi) QC and standardisation, (xii) clinical evaluation, etc. (Mukherjee *et al.*, 2014b). Traditional use of medicinal plants needs to be systematically investigated and standardised with respect to quality, safety and efficacy Macroscopic and microscopic studies, genetic fingerprinting methods, analytical chemical fingerprinting techniques e.g. high performance liquid chromatography (HPLC), high performance thin layer chromatography (HPTLC), capillary electrophoresis (CE), or gas chromatography LC-MS/MS are preferred tools for standardisation. Although there has been an increase in interest in science-based research into herbal medicine, some of the research to date has been overwhelmed by studies conducted using unauthenticated and uncharacterised products (Mukherjee *et al.*, 2014a; Patra *et al.*, 2010).

In reverse pharmacology, researchers start with the final product, a clinically useful compound for example, and work backwards to find out what it contains and how it functions. This can offer clues about how particular medicines work, and where they act in the body. High-throughput screening is the advanced screening technology that relies on high-speed data processing and sensitive detectors to conduct millions of biochemical, genetic or pharmacological tests in a few minutes. The process can quickly identify active compounds that affect particular biological pathways. Systems biology deals with the holistic approach to know different chemicals and metabolic processes to interact within the body. Since TMs often have numerous active ingredients, it could be used to measure the whole body's response to the mixture of compounds (Patwardhan and Mashelka, 2009).

Metabolomics study reveals to the quantitative and qualitative estimation of "whole-set of metabolites" formed in a cellular/organism system. It may be defined as the systemic study of the individual chemical fingerprints that definite cellular process leaves behind and even more particularly, the technique of the metabolite profile of molecules in an organism. The combined data of all the metabolites in a biological system, which are the final products of its gene expression, is known as metabolome. These approaches deal with the study of genomics, transcriptomics and proteomics of biological systems (Heyman and Meyer, 2012).

Herbal medicine are complex products because a single medicinal plant constitutes hundreds of phyto-constituents and their pharmacological properties are influenced by the time of collection, area of plant origin, and environmental conditions, so special attention is needed for its cultivation and collection for quality of products. Therefore, the above mentioned strategies regarding various issues are needed for validation of TM (Mukherjee and Houghton, 2009).

6.5 Chemical Profiling and Standardisation of Indian Traditional Medicine

Chemical profiling of traditional herbal preparations is essential in order to assess the quality of drugs. It deals with bioactive compound quantification, spurious drug determination, comparative fingerprint analysis, standardisation of herbs, stability of formulations and quality consistency of TMPs (Mukherjee *et al.*, 2012). Botanicals are mostly obtained from wild sources and have the greatest challenges for ensuring consistent product quality (Mukherjee *et al.*, 2011). There are so many environmental factors including soil conditions, availability of light and water, temperature variations, nutrients and geographical location affect the phytoconstituents present in plants. Further cultivation and harvesting techniques and storage methods also influence the physical appearance and chemical constituents of the plant. This means quality parameters should be set not only for the plant materials but also for plant extracts and final product. Botanical extracts made directly from crude plant material show substantial variation in composition, quality and therapeutic effects. The standardisation of herbal drugs includes authentication, harvesting the best quality raw material, assessment of intermediate, finished product. As the genetic composition is unique for each species and is not affected by age, physiological conditions and environmental factors. DNA-based markers are also used in the identification of inter/intra-species variation (Mukherjee *et al.*, 2013a).

Standardised extracts are high-quality extracts containing consistent levels of specified compounds and they are subjected to rigorous QCs during all phases of the growing, harvesting, and manufacturing processes. When the active principles are unknown, marker substance should be established for analytical purposes and standardisation. Marker substances are chemically defined constituents of herbal drug that are important for the quality of the finished product. Ideally, the chemical markers chosen should be bioactive (Mukherjee and Verpoorte, 2003).

Marker compound selection is generally based upon a variety of different factors including stability, ease of analysis, time and cost of analysis, relevance to therapeutic effect and indicator of product quality or stability. Various chemical markers have been described for the validation of TM including therapeutic components, bioactive components, synergistic components, characteristic components, main component, correlative components, toxic components and general components. Indian Council of Medical Research has published three volumes on "Phytochemical Reference Standards of Indian Medicinal Plants". As discussed in the monographs of the American Herbal Pharmacopoeia (AHP), the use of single or multiple chemical markers was important to QC apart from proper cultivation, collection and quality, optimum extraction and standardisation of raw materials, the evaluation of herbal medicine should be done in better way to get fruitful results (Mukherjee *et al.*, 2010a, 2011).

Chemical fingerprints can be used to authenticate plant material, identification and quantification of active compounds to relate the chemical composition to biological activity for product standardisation and validation (Mukherjee *et al.*, 2012). Chemical markers are frequently used for assuring quality consistency of natural products derived from botanical sources. Marker compounds are not necessarily pharmacologically active all the time but their presence is well established in products with characteristic chemical features (Mukherjee *et al.*, 2013a). Marker components may be classified as active principles, active markers and analytical makers, while biomarkers may be defined as pharmacologicalled active. Usually, determination of single or several marker compounds by a developed method is required for QC purpose. Marker-based standards are becoming popular for the identification/authentication of herbal drug components (Mukherjee *et al.*, 2007, 2011).

Quality of TMPs can be defined as the status of a drug that is determined by identity, purity, content, physical and biological properties. QC is very importance for efficacy and safety of herbal products. QC for herbal medicine begins from the field and ends with a safe and effective product being delivered to the patient, followed by post-marketing pharmacovigilance. WHO has developed a series of technical guidelines and documents relating to the safety and QA of medicinal plants and herbal materials. To develop quality herbal product good practices including Good Agriculture Practices (GAP), Good Harvesting Practices (GHP), Good Storage Practices (GSP), Good Clinical Practice (GCP), Good Manufacturing Practices (GMP) and Good Laboratory Practices (GLP) (Mukherjee and Houghton, 2004) are essential to follow. Table 6.2. gives important chemical constituent of medicinal plants commonly used in Ayurveda and other ISM.

6.5.1 *Plant Metabolomics*

Metabolomics has become a powerful tool in drug discovery and development by identification and profiling of secondary metabolites from natural resources (Harrigan and Goodacre, 2003). Medicinal plant-based metabolomics study is of prime importance, as there are more than 200,000 plant secondary metabolites, which have been reported from natural resources (Trethewey, 2004). There are several well-known cancer chemotherapeutic drugs derived from plant secondary metabolites, such as paclitaxel (taxol), camptothecin (irinotecan and topotecan), and podophyllotoxins (etoposide and teniposide). The great potential of plant secondary metabolites or natural products to serve as health care products or lead compounds for new drug development have renewed interest in pharmaceutical and nutraceutical research (Newman and Cragg, 2007). The use of whole plants or extracts as medicines gave way to the isolation of active compounds, beginning in the early 19th century with the isolation of morphine from opium.

A study involved in the characterisation of a set of defined metabolites is known as "targeted" metabolomics and usually combines NMR-MS techniques, which is applied for such type of analysis (Dudley *et al.*, 2010). Thousands of metabolites can be detected by this method in a single elute and it is the global approach that is leading the way to major revelation in our understanding of cell biology, physiology and medicine (Cox *et al.*, 2014). Metabolomics study has diverse fields of application and can be divided into four areas: (i) target compound analysis — the quantification of specific metabolites, (ii) the metabolomic profiling — the quantitative

Table 6.2. Important bioactive compounds discovered from Indian TM.

Traditional medicine	Parts used	Active constituents	Biological activity
Allium sativum (Banerjee *et al.*, 2003)	Bulb	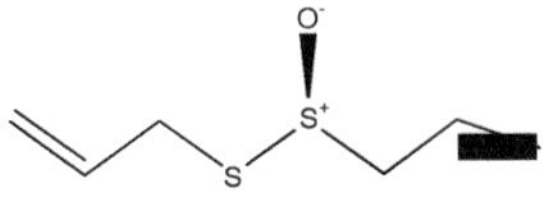 Allicin	Hypolipidaemic, anti-atherosclerotic, hypoglycaemic, anti-coagulant, anti-hypertensive, anti-microbial, anti-cancer, antidote (for heavy metal poisoning), hepatoprotective and immunomodulatory
Aloe vera (Mukherjee *et al.*, 2014a)	Leave (gel)	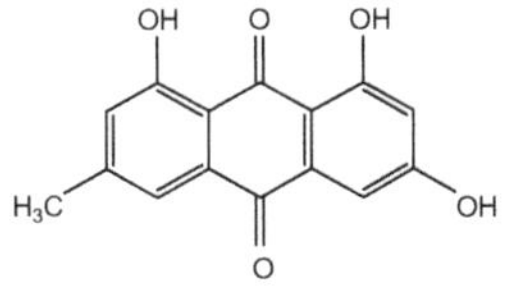 Emodin	Wound healing, Anti-inflammatory, anti-fungal, hypoglycemic and gastroprotective
Andrographis paniculata (Maiti *et al.*, 2010)	Leave	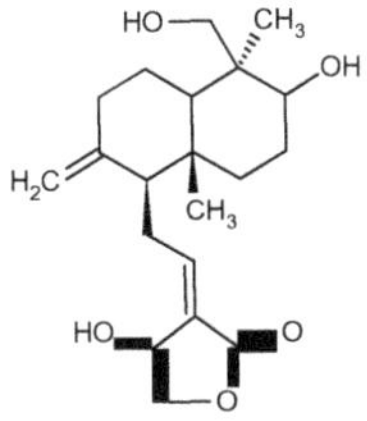 Andrographolide	Treatment of fever, inflammation, common cold, upper respiratory tract infection, tonsillitis, pharyngitis, laryngitis, pneumonia, tuberculosis, pyelonephritis and hepatic disorder
Bacopa monnieri (Ganzera *et al.*, 2004)	Whole plant	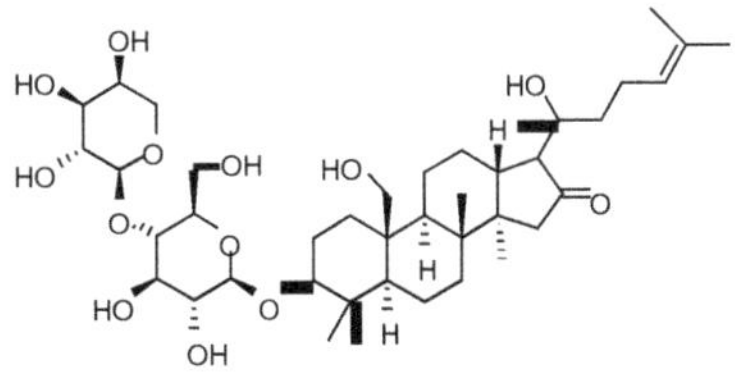 Bacoside	Used as memory enhancer, brain tonic, anti-asthmatic and antipyretic

(Continued)

Table 6.2. (*Continued*)

Traditional medicine	Parts used	Active constituents	Biological activity
Boswellia serrata (Hüsch *et al.*, 2013)	Gum resin	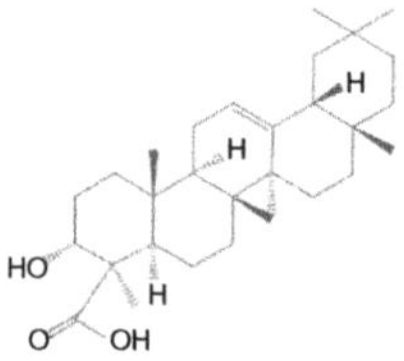 Boswellic acids	Used in inflammatory bowel disease, rheumatoid arthritis, osteoarthritis and asthma
Calendula officinalis (Fonseca *et al.*, 2011)	Flower	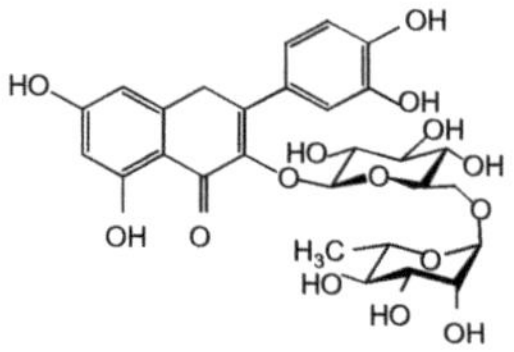 Rutin	anti-inflammatory, anti-oxidant, wound healing, UV-screening, anti-aging and anti-mutagenic
Camellia sinensis (Chatterjee *et al.*, 2012)	Leave	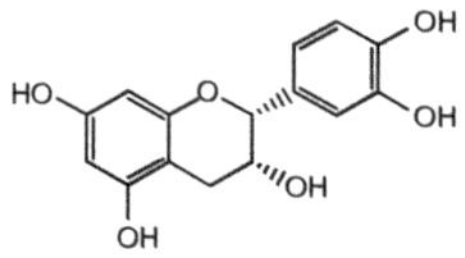 Epicatechin	Anti-ageing, anti-diabetic, neuroprotective, anti-mutagenicity, anti-obesity, anti-bacterial and anti-HIV
Capsicum annuum (Gantait *et al.*, 2010)	Fruit	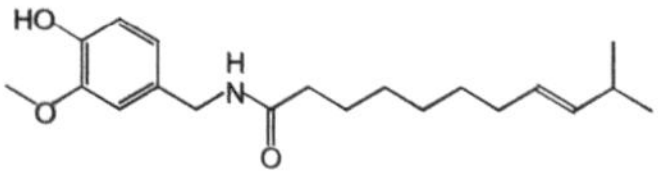 Capsaicin	Analgesic, counterirritant, rheumatism, lumbago, neuralgia, to treat hoarseness, atonicdyspepsia, loss of appetite and flatulence
Centella asiatica (Nema *et al.*, 2013)	Leave	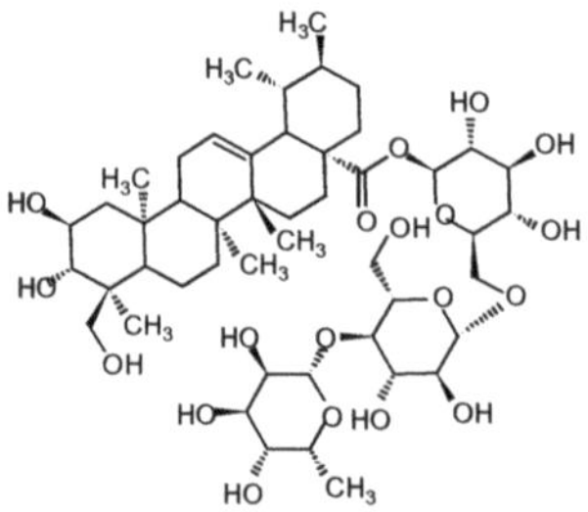 Asiaticoside	Anti-wrinkle, used in wound healing and anti-histimincs

(*Continued*)

Table 6.2. (*Continued*)

Traditional medicine	Parts used	Active constituents	Biological activity
Coffea arabica (Zhang *et al.*, 2010)	Seed	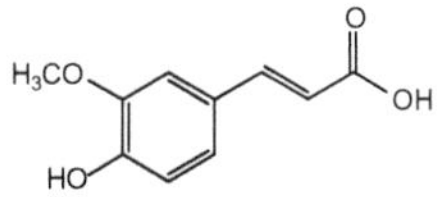 Ferulic acid	Anti-oxidant, antiageing, hepatoprotective, anti-atherogenic, anti-mutagenic, anti-inflammatory, anti-cancer, anti-diabetic, neuroprotective and cardio-protective activities
Crocus sativus (Das *et al.*, 2004)	Flowering tops	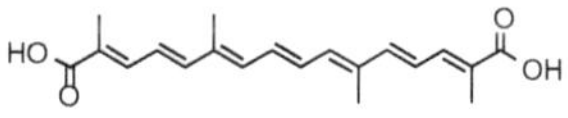 Crocetin	Potent anti-oxidant, anti-cancer and photoprotectant
Curcuma longa (Gantait *et al.*, 2011)	Rhizome	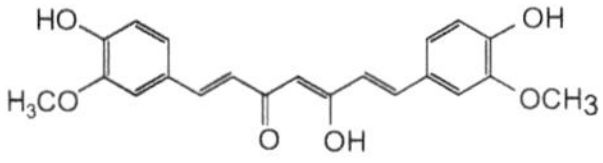 Curcumin	Anti-tumour, anti-oxidant, anti-arthritic, anti-amyloid, Anti-ischemic and antiinflam-matory
Emblica officinalis (Ponnusankar *et al.*, 2011a, 2011b)	Fruit	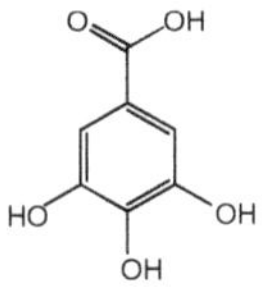 Gallic acid	Hepatoprotective, anti-oxidant, anti-diabetic, anti-tumor and immunomo-dulatory
Eugenia caryophyllata (Gopu *et al.*, 2008)	Flower bud	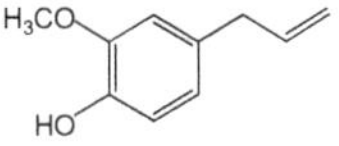 Eugenol	Anti-inflammatory, anti-oxidant, carminative, anti-spasmodic, anti-septic and anti-microbial agent

(*Continued*)

Table 6.2. (*Continued*)

Traditional medicine	Parts used	Active constituents	Biological activity
Gingko biloba (Bhattaram *et al.*, 2002)	Leave	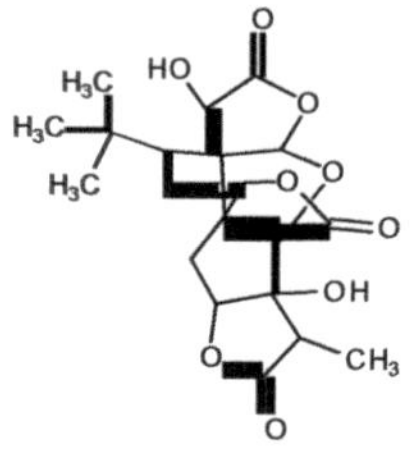 Ginkgolide A 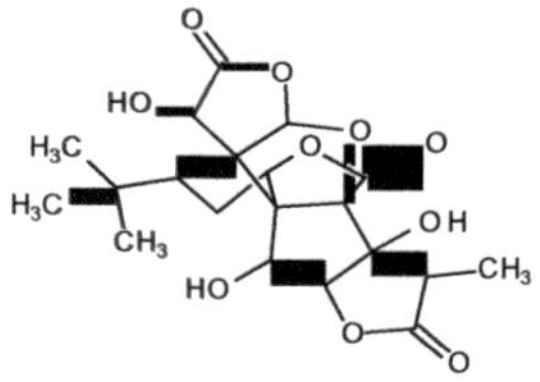 Ginkgolide B	Used in peripheral circulatory insufficiency, cerebrovascular disorders, geriatric complaints alzheimer dementia, anti-oxidant and anti-cancer
Glycine max (Afaq and Mukhtar, 2006)	Seed	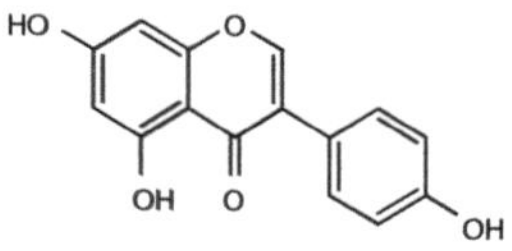 Genistein	Anti-oxidant, anti-carcinogenic and anti-aging
Glycyrrhiza glabra (Harwansh *et al.*, 2011)	Root and rhizome	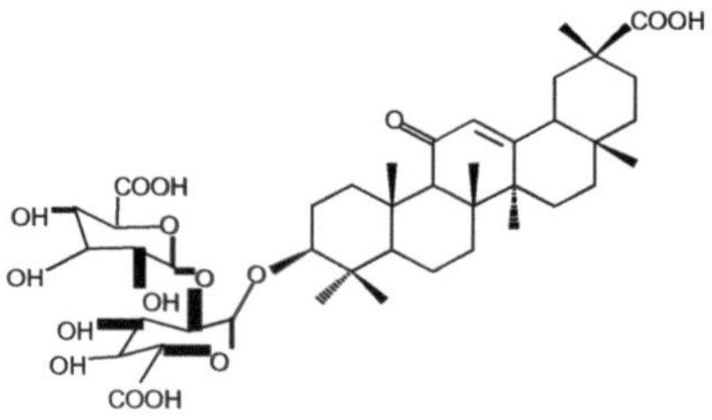 Glycyrrhizin	Anti-inflammatory and anti-ulcer, hepatoprotective, anti-allergic, anti-arthritic, anti-arrhythmic, anti-bacterial, anti-viral and anti-asthmatic

(*Continued*)

Table 6.2. (*Continued*)

Traditional medicine	Parts used	Active constituents	Biological activity
Hypericum perforatum (Bhattaram *et al.*, 2002)	Aerial parts	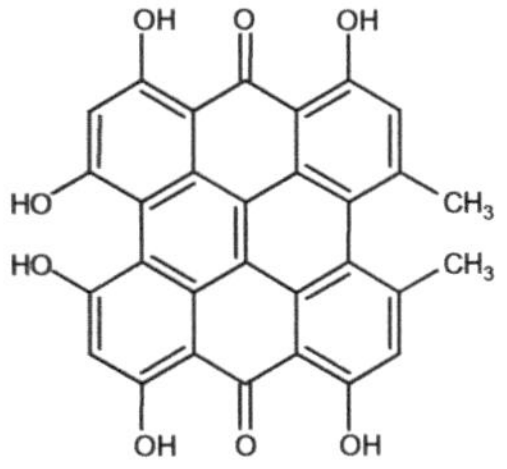 Hypericin	Anti-depressants, anti-microbial, anti-fungal and other CNS disorder
Nelumbo nucifera (Mukherjee *et al.*, 2010)	Rhizome	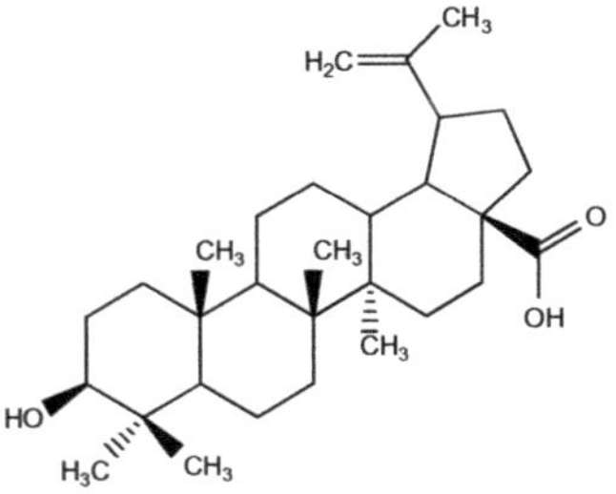 Betulinic acid	Used in pharyngopathy, pectoralgia, leukoderma, strangury, dysentery, cough, hematemesis, tissue inflammation, cancer, skin diseases and diabetes
Ocimum sanctum (The Ayurvedic pharmacopoeia of India, 2001)	Leave	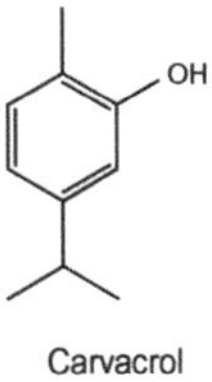 Carvacrol	Anti-oxidant, anti-bacterial anti-hypertensive and to treat respiratory complications
Piper longum and *Piper nigrum* (Harwansh *et al.*, 2014)	Fruit	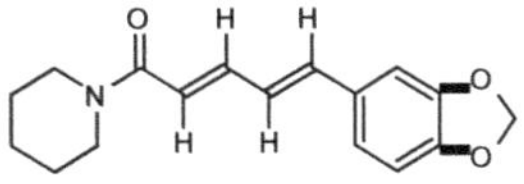 Piperine	Anti-ageing, revitalising, memory enhancing, adaptogenic, anti-diarrhoeal, anti-spasmodic, immunomodulatory, remedies for cough, cold, fever, asthma and other respiratory problems

(*Continued*)

Table 6.2. (*Continued*)

Traditional medicine	Parts used	Active constituents	Biological activity
Punica granatum (Afaq and Mukhtar, 2006)	Fruit	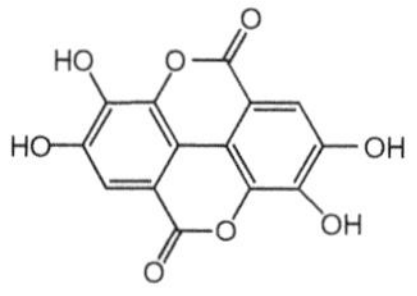 Ellagic acid	Anti-oxidant, anti-aging and anti-inflammatory
Silybum marianum (Bhattaram *et al.*, 2002)	Fruit	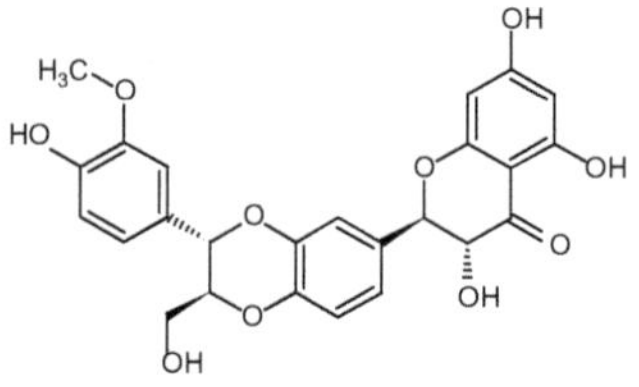	Used in a whole range of liver and gall bladder conditions including hepatitis and cirrhosis. Anti-oxidant, anti-carcinogenic and anti-inflammatory
Terminalia belerica (Ponnusankar *et al.*, 2011a) and *Terminalia chebula* (Ponnusankar *et al.*, 2011b)	Fruit	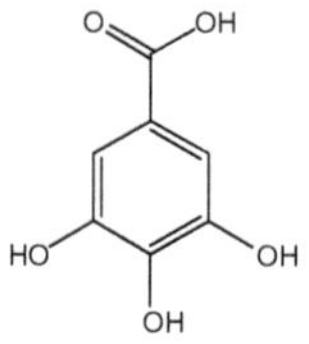 Gallic acid	Anti-atherosclerotic, hepatoprotective, cardioprotective, cytoprotective, cardiotonic, anti-mutagenic and anti-fungal
Zingiber officinale (Harwansh *et al.*, 2014)	Rhizome	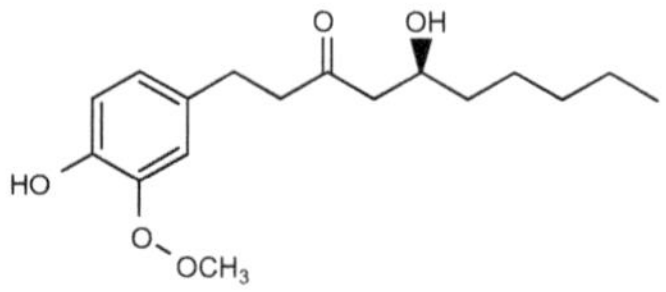 Gingerol	Anti-viral (hRSV), anti-inflammatory, bronchitis and other respiratory tract infections

and qualitative estimation of a set compounds, (iii) metabolite chemo-analysis — the qualitative and quantitative analysis of all metabolites and (iv) metabolomic fingerprinting — sample classification by rapid global analysis (Merzenich *et al.*, 2014). These approaches emphasised the phyto medicine research that may assist evidence-based phyto-therapeutics, and such research may lead to a change of paradigm in the development and application of multicomponent botanical therapeutics (MCBT) (Hu and Xu, 2014).

Chemo profiling of the metabolites can help to identify the metabolites and to compare the nature of compounds. The output of sensors (analytical detectors) is known as "profiling" which are classified and statistically analysed to marks out their differences (Noteborn *et al.*, 2000). It involves identification of metabolites as the analysis is based on their spectral peaks and calibration curves. Metabolome investigation comprehensively examines entire range of metabolites in a sample by the mutual application of various analytical techniques (Glassbrook and Ryals, 2001). Metabolomics allows an overall calculation of a cellular system, in regards to the gene regulation, modulated enzyme kinetics and variations in metabolic reactions. In difference to the genomics or proteomics, metabolomics reveals the phenotypic changes in the function (Harrigan and Goodacre, 2013). However, it is important to mention here that the "omic" sciences are corresponding as "upstream" changes in genes and proteins are considered as changes "downstream" in physiological function. The divergent of metabolomics is that it is a terminal view of the biological system, not allowing for demonstration of the increased or decreased genes and proteins (Gahlaut *et al.*, 2012). The markers used for the standardisation, chemical and DNA fingerprinting, bioassays, metabolomics approach and the emerging field of phytomics provide mechanisms for assuring consistent quality and efficacy of herbal medicine (Mukherjee *et al.*, 2013a). Several Indian TMs such as *Curcuma longa*, *Boerrhaevia diffusa*, *Glycyrrhiza glabra*, *Echinacea angustifolia*, *Saraca asoca*, *Withania somnifera*, *Psoralea corylifolia*, *Zanthoxylum armatum*, *Tinospora cordifolia* and *Commiphora wightii* have been established for the different therapeutic activities and their metabolite profiling, which has been described in Table 6.3.

6.6 Conclusion

Medicinal plants are not only a major resource base for the TM and herbal industry but also provide livelihood and health security to a large segment of Indian population. Ministry of AYUSH, Government of India has taken several initiatives for promotion and development of TM.

Table 6.3. Metabolite fingerprinting of some Indian traditional medicinal plants.

Medicinal plant	Metabolomics approach	Metabolites
Curcuma longa (Jiang *et al.*, 2006)	LC-ESI-MS/MS	Curcumin; Demethoxycurcumin; Bisdemethoxycurcumin; 1,7-Bis(4- hydroxyphenyl)-3,5-heptanediol; 5-Hydroxy-1,7-bis(4-hydroxyphenyl)-3- heptanone; 1,7-Bis(4-hydroxy-3-methoxyphenyl)-4,6-heptadien-3-one; 1-(4-Hydroxy-3-methoxyphenyl)-7-(4-hydroxy-3,5-dimethoxyphenyl)-4,6-heptadien-3-one; 5-Hydroxy-1,7-bis(3,4-dihydroxyphenyl)-1-hepten-3-one; 4-Hydroxybisdemethoxycurcumin
Boerrhaevia diffusa (Pereira *et al.*, 2009)	HS-SPME-GC-MS	Phellandrene; a-Pinene; 3 Limonene; Camphor; Isomenthone; Menthol; Geranylacetone; cis 4-Hexen-1-ol; trans 2-Octanal; 2-Nonen-1-ol; 2- Decen-1-ol; Methylpyrrole; 3-Phenyl-2-(20-pyridyl)-indole; Eugenol; Vanilin; β-Cyclocitral; β-Ionone; Dihydroactinidiolide; Linalyl anthranilate; 4-Oxoisophorone; Resorcinol monoacetate; Benzothiazol; Benzophenone
Glycyrrhiza species (*Glycyrrhiza glabra, Glycyrrhiza uralensis, Glycyrrhiza inflata* and *Glycyrrhiza echinata*) (Farag *et al.*, 2012)	1H NMR, GC-MS , LC-MS and PCA	Glycyrrhizin; Sucrose; Liquiritin; Isoliquiritin; Liquiritigenin; Isoliquiritigenin; 4-Hydroxyphenyl acetic acid; Licochalcone; Rhamnose (glycosides)
Echinacea species (*Echinacea purpurea, Echinacea pallida* and *Echinacea angustifolia*) (Hou *et al.*, 2010)	HPLC/ESI/MS, GAP, Biplot	Undeca-2Z(E),4E(Z)-dien-8,10-diynoic acid- isobutylamide; Trideca-2E,7Z- dien-10,12-diynoic acid-isobutylamide; Dodeca-2Z,4E-dien-8,10-diynoic acid-isobutylamide; Dodeca-2E,4Z-dien-8,10-diynoic acid-isobutylamide; Dodeca-2E,4E,8Z-trienoic acid-isobutylamide; Undeca-2E(Z)-en-8,10- diynoic acid- isobutylamide; Dodeca-2E-en-8,10-diynoic acid- isobutylamide; Undeca-2Z-en-8,10-diynoic acid- 2-methylbutylamide; Dodeca-2E-en-8,10-diynoic acid-2 methylbutylamide; Pentadeca-2E,9Z- dien-12,14-diynoic acid-isobutylamide; Pentadeca-1,8-diene; pentadeca-1,8,11-trien; Heptadeca-1,8,11-triene; Pentadeca-8Z-en-2-one; Pentadeca-8Z,11Z-dien; Pentadeca-8Z-en-11,13-diyn-2-one; Aromadendren; Germacrene-D; γ-Gurjunene; p-Menth-1-ene-6-ol

Saraca asoca (Gahlaut *et al.*, 2013)	UPLC-QTOFMS	(R) Prunasin; Sn-Glycero-3-phosphocholine; Delphinidin; O-Phosphocholine; Procyanidin B1; (-) Epicatechin
Withania somnifera (Chatterjee *et al.*, 2010)	GC-MS, HPLC and NMR	Palmitic acid; Oleic acid; Linoleic acid; Linolenic acid; Citric acid; Fructose-5 TMS; Fructose-5 TMS, Fructose-5 TMS, Fumaric acid (L); GABA (L & R); Galactose (L & R); Glycerol (R); Glutamate (L & R); 2 O-Glutamine (L & R); a-Glucose (L & R); b-Glucose (L & R); Glycine (L); Myo-inositol (L); Isoleucine (L); Lactic acid; Lysine; Leucine (L); Succinate (L & R); Malic acid 3 TMS; N-Acetyl-Glucosamine (L); Phenyl alanine (L); Tartaric acid (L); Benzoic acid (L & R); Butandioic acid (L); Phenyl acetic acid (L & R); p- Hydroxy, phenyl ethanol (L); p-Hydroxy, phenyl acetic acid (R); 3,4,5- Trihydroxy cinnamic acid (R); β-Sitosterol (L)
Psoralea corylifolia (Abhyankar *et al.*, 2005)	GC/MS, HPLC/UV–MS	Psoralene; Stigmasta-5-en-3-ol; Stigmasta-5,22-dien-3-ol; Daidzein; Neophytadiene; 2-Furancarboxaldehyde,5-(hydroxymethyl); Myristic acid; Caryophyllene oxide; Phytol; Bakuchiol; 1,2-Benzenedicarboxylic acid; 2,6-Dimethoxyphenol; 2,8-Diisopropyl-peri-xanthenoxanthene-4,10-quinone; Linoleic acid; Palmitic acid; Stearic acid; 1-Eicosanol
Zanthoxylum armatum (Kumar *et al.*, 2014)	UPLC-DAD-ESI-QTOF-MS/MS	Rubemamin; Zanthosin; N-(4-methoxy-phenethyl)-3,4-dimethoxy- cinnamamide; Eudesmin; Magnolin or epimagnolin; Isomer of hydroxy- sanshool; Armatamide; Horsfieldin; Hydroxy-α-sanshool; Isomer of hydroxy-sanshool; Xanthoxylin; Dioxamin; Kobusin; Fargesin; Sesamin; Asarinin
Tinospora cordifolia (Shirolkar *et al.*, 2013)	UPLC-QTOFMS	Jatrorrhizine; Mangoflorine; Menisperine; Columbamine; Berberine; Tinosporoside
Commiphora wightii (Bhatia *et al.*, 2015)	NMR, GC–MS, HPLC	Guggulsterone E and Z; D-limonene; β-Myrcene; α-Caryophyllene; β-Caryophyllene; δ-Cadiene; β-Elemene; Guaiacol; Isoeugenol; Verticiol; Quinic acid; myo-Inositol; α-Tocopherol; n-Methylpyrrolidone; trans- Farnesol; Prostaglandin F2; Protocatechuic; Gallic acid; Cinnamic acids

Acknowledgement

The authors are thankful to the Department of Biotechnology, Government of India, New Delhi, for financial support through Tata Innovation Fellowship (D.O. No. BT/HRD/35/01/04/2014) to PKM.

References

Abhyankar, G., Reddy, V.D., Giri, C.C., Rao, K.V., Lakshmi, V.V.S., Prabhakar, S., Vairamani, M., Thippeswamy, B.S. and Bhattacharya, P.S. (2005). Amplified fragment length polymorphism and metabolomics profiles of hairy roots of *Psoralea corylifolia* L. *Phytochemistry* **66**, 2441–2457.

Afaq, F. and Mukhtar, H. (2006). Botanical antioxidants in the prevention of photocarcinogenesis and photoaging. *Exp. Dermatol.* **15**, 678–684.

Anonymous (2001). *Caraka Samhita-Sharira Sthanam.* Chaukhamba Sanskrit Series Office, Varanasi.

AYUSH (2015). AYUSH in India, Planning & Evaluation Cell, Department of Ayurveda, Yoga & Naturopathy, Unani, Siddha and Homoeopathy (AYUSH). Ministry of Health and Family Welfare, Government of India.

Banerjee, S.K., Mukherjee, P.K. and Maulik, S.K. (2003). Garlic as an antioxidant: the good, the bad and the ugly. *Phytother. Res.* **17**, 97–106.

Bhatia, A., Bharti, S.K., Tripathi, T., Mishra, A., Sidhu, O.P., Roy, R. and Nautiyal, C.S. (2015). Metabolic profiling of *Commiphora wightii* (guggul) reveals a potential source for pharmaceuticals and nutraceuticals. *Phytochemistry* **110**, 29–36.

Bhattaram, V.A., Graefe, U., Kohlert, C., Veit, M. and Derendorf, H. (2002). Pharmacokinetics and bioavailability of herbal medicinal products. *Phytomedicine* **9**, 1–33.

Chatterjee, S., Srivastava, S., Khalid, A., Singh, N., Sangwan, R.S., Sidhu, O.P., Roy, R., Khetrapal, C.L. and Tuli, R. (2010). Comprehensive metabolic fingerprinting of *Withania somnifera* leaf and root extracts. *Phytochemistry* **71**, 1085–1094.

Chatterjee, P., Chandra, S., Dey, P. and Bhattacharya, S. (2012). Evaluation of anti-inflammatory effects of green tea and black tea: a comparative in vitro study. *J. Adv. Pharm. Technol. Res.* **3**, 136–138.

Cordell, G.A. and Colvard, M.D. (2012). Natural products and traditional medicine: turning on a paradigm. *J. Nat. Prod.* **75**, 514–525.

Cox, D.G., Oh, J., Keasling, A., Colson, K. and Hamann, M.T. (2014). The utility of metabolomics in natural product and biomarker characterization. *Biochim. Biophys. Acta* **1840**, 3460–3474.

Das, I., Chakrabarty, R.N. and Das, S. (2004). Saffron can prevent chemically induced skin carcinogenesis in Swiss albino mice. *Asian Pac. J. Cancer Prev.* **5**(1), 70–76.

Debnath, P.K., Banerjee, S., Debnath, P., Mitra, A. and Mukherjee, P.K. (2015). Ayurveda — opportunities for developing safe and effective treatment choices for the future. In: *Evidence-Based Validation of Herbal Medicine*, Mukherjee PK. (Ed.), 1st Edition, Elsevier, Amsterdam.

Dudley, E., Yousef, M., Wang, Y. and Griffiths, W. (2010). Targeted metabolomics and mass spectrometry. *Adv. Protein Chem. Struct. Biol.* **80**, 45–83.

Farag, M.A., Porzel, A. and Wessjohann, L.A. (2012). Comparative metabolite profiling and fingerprinting of medicinal licorice roots using a multiplex approach of GC-MS, LC-MS and 1D NMR techniques. *Phytochemistry* **76**, 60–72.

Fonseca, Y.M., Catini, C.D., Vicentini, F.T.M.C., Cardoso, J.C., Junior, R.L.C.A. and Fonseca, M.J.V. (2011). Efficacy of marigold extract-loaded formulations against UV-induced oxidative stress. *J. Pharm. Sci.* **100**(6), 2182–2193.

Gahlaut, A., Taneja, P., Shirolkar, A., Nale, A., Hooda, V. and Dabur, R. (2012). Principal component and partial least square discriminant based analysis of methanol extracts of bark and regenerated bark of *Saraca asoca*. *Int. J. Pharm. Pharm. Sci.* **4**, 331–335.

Gahlaut, A., Shirolkar, A., Hooda, V. and Dabur, R. (2013). A rapid and simple approach to discriminate various extracts of *Saraca asoca* [Roxb.], De. Wild using UPLC-QTOFMS and multivariate analysis. *J. Pharm. Res.* **7**, 143–149.

Gantait, A., Pandit, S., Nema, N. and Mukherjee, P.K. (2010). Quantification of glycyrrhizin in *Glycyrrhiza glabra* extract by validated HPTLC densitometry. *J. AOAC Int.* **93**, 492–495.

Gantait, A., Barman, T. and Mukherjee, P.K. (2011). Validated method for estimation of curcumin in turmeric powder. *Indian J. Tradit. Knowle.* **10**(2), 247–250.

Ganzera, M., Gampenrieder, J., Pawar, R.S., Khan, I.A. and Stuppner, H. (2004). Separation of the major triterpenoid saponins in *Bacopa monnieri* by high-performance liquid chromatography. *Anal. Chim. Acta* **516**, 149–154.

Glassbrook, N. and Ryals, J.A. (2001). Systematic approach to biochemical profiling. *Curr. Opin. Plant Biol.* **4**, 186–190.

Gopu, C.L., Aher, S., Mehta, H., Paradkar, A.R. and Mahadik, K.R. (2008). Simultaneous determination of cinnamaldehyde, eugenol and piperine by HPTLC densitometric method. *Phytochem. Anal.* **19**, 116–121.

Harrigan, G.G. and Goodacre, R. (2003). *Metabolic Profiling: It's Role in Biomarker Discovery and Gene Function Analysis.* Kluwer Academic Publishers, Boston.

Harwansh, R.K., Patra, K.C., Pareta, S.K., Singh, J., and Biswas, R. (2011). Pharmacological studies of *Glycyrrhiza glabra*: a review. *Pharmacologyonline* **2**, 1032–1038.

Harwansh, R.K., Mukherjee, K., Bhadra, S., Kar, A., Bahadur, S., Mitra, A. and Mukherjee, P.K. (2014). Cytochrome P450 inhibitory potential and RP-HPLC standardization of *trikatu*-a rasayana from Indian ayurveda. *J. Ethnopharmacol.* **153**, 674–681.

Heyman, H.M. and Meyer, J.J.M. (2012). NMR-based metabolomics as a quality control tool for herbal products. *S. Afr. J. Bot.* **82**, 21–32.

Hou, C.C., Chen, C.H., Yang, N.S., Chen, Y.P., Lo, C.P., Wang, S.Y., Tien, Y.J., Tsai, P.W. and Shyur, L.F. (2010). Comparative metabolomics approach coupled with cell- and gene-based assays for species classification and anti-inflammatory bioactivity validation of Echinacea plants. *J. Nutr. Biochem.* **21**, 1045–1059.

Hu, C. and Xu, G. (2014). Metabolomics and traditional Chinese medicine. *Trends Anal. Chem.* **61**, 207–214.

Hüsch, J., Bohnet, J., Fricker, G., Skarke, C., Artaria, C., Appendino, G. *et al.* (2013). Enhanced absorption of boswellic acids by a lecithin delivery form (Phytosome®) of Boswellia extract. *Fitoterapia* **84**, 89–98.

Jiang, H., Timmermann, B.N. and Gang, D.R. (2006). Use of liquid chromatography–electrospray ionization tandem mass spectrometry to identify diaryl-heptanoids in turmeric (*Curcuma longa* L.) rhizome. *J. Chromatogr. A* **1111**, 21–31.

Katiyar, C., Gupta, A., Kanjilal, S. and Katiyar, S. (2012). Drug discovery from plant sources: an integrated approach. *Ayurveda* **33**(1), 10–19.

Kumar, V., Kumar, S., Singh, B. and Kumar, N. (2014). Quantitative and structural analysis of amides and lignans in *Zanthoxylum armatum* by UPLC-DAD-ESI-QTOF-MS/MS. *J. Pharm. Biomed. Anal.* **94**, 23–29.

Li, S., Han, Q., Qiao, C., Song, J., Cheng, C.L. and Xu, H. (2008). Chemical markers for the quality control of herbal medicines: an overview. *Chinese Medicine* **3**(7), 1–16.

Maiti, K., Mukherjee, K., Murugan, V., Saha, B.P. and Mukherjee, P.K. (2010). Enhancing bioavailability and hepatoprotective activity of andrographolide from *Andrographis paniculata*, a well-known medicinal food, through its herbosome. *J. Sci. Food. Agric.* **90**, 43–51.

Mukherjee, P.K. (2001). Evaluation of Indian traditional medicine. *Drug Inf. J.* **35**, 631–640.

Mukherjee, P.K. and Verpoorte, R. (2003). *GMP for Botanicals-Regulatory and Quality Issues on Phytomedicines.* 1st Edition. Business Horizons, New Delhi.

Mukherjee, P.K. and Wahile, A. (2006). Integrated approaches towards drug development from Ayurveda and other Indian system of medicines. *J. Ethnopharmacol.* **103**, 25–35.

Mukherjee, P.K., Rai, S., Kumar, V., Mukherjee, K., Hyland, P.J. and Hider, R.C. (2007). Plants of Indian origin in drug discovery. *Expert Opin. Drug Discov.* **2**(5), 633–657.

Mukherjee, P.K. and Houghton, P.J. (2009). The worldwide phenomenon of increased use of herbal products: opportunity and threats. In: *Evaluation of Herbal Medicinal Products–Perspectives on Quality, Safety and Efficacy*, 1st Edition. Pharmaceutical Press, Great Britain.

Mukherjee, D., Kumar, N.S., Khatua, T. and Mukherjee, P.K. (2010a). Rapid validated HPTLC method for estimation of betulinic acid in *Nelumbo nucifera* (Nymphaeaceae) rhizome extract. *Phytochem. Anal.* **21**, 556–560.

Mukherjee, P.K., Venkatesh, P. and Ponnusankar, S. (2010b). Ethnopharmacology and integrative medicine – let the history tell the future. *J. Ayurveda Integr. Med.* **1**(2), 100–109.

Mukherjee, P.K., Ponnusankar, S., Venkatesh, P., Gantait, A. and Pal, B.C. (2011). Marker profiling: an approach for quality evaluation of Indian medicinal plants. *Drug Inf. J.* **45**, 1–14.

Mukherjee, P.K., Nema, N.K., Venkatesh, P. and Debnath, P.K. (2012). Changing scenario for promotion and development of Ayurveda — way forward. *J. Ethnopharmacol.* **143**, 424–434.

Mukherjee, P.K., Harwansh, R.K. and Bahadur, S. (2013a). Standardization and chemo-profiling of herbal medicine through marker analysis. *The Pharma Review* 51–58.

Mukherjee, P.K., Bahadur, S., Harwansh, R.K., Nema, N.K. and Bhadra, S. (2013b). Development of traditional medicines: globalizing local knowledge or localizing global technologies. *Pharma Times* **45**, 39–42.

Mukherjee, P.K., Bahadur, S., Harwansh, R.K. and Chaudhary, S.K. (2014a). Shifting paradigm for validation of medicinal plants in Indian traditional medicine. *Indian Drugs* **51**(8), 5–14.

Mukherjee, P.K., Nema, N.K., Maity, N., Mukherjee, K. and Harwansh, R.K. (2014b). Phytochemical and therapeutic profile of *Aloe vera. J. Nat. Remedies* **14**(1), 1–26.

Narayana, D.B.A., Katayar, C.K. and Brindavanam, N.B. (1998). Original system: search, research or re-search. *IDMA Bulletin* **29**, 413–416.

Nema, N.K., Dalai, M.K. and Mukherjee, P.K. (2011). Ayush herbs and status que in herbal industries. *The Pharma Review* 141–148.

Nema, N.K., Maity, N., Sarkar, B.K. and Mukherjee, P.K. (2013). Matrix metalloproteinase, hyaluronidase and elastase inhibitory potential of standardized extract of *Centella asiatica. Pharm. Biol.* **51**(9), 1182–1187.

Newman, D.J. and Cragg, G.M. (2007). Natural products as sources of new drugs over the last 25 years. *J. Nat. Prod.* **70**, 461–477.

Noteborn, H.P., Lommen, A., Van-Jagt, R.C. and Weseman, J.M. (2000). Chemical fingerprinting for the evaluation of unintended secondary metabolic changes in transgenic food crops. *J. Biotechnol.* **77**, 103–114.

Patra, K.C., Pareta, S.K., Harwansh, R.K. and Kumar, K.J. (2010). Traditional approaches towards standardization of herbal medicines – a review. *J. Pharm. Sci. Technol.* **2**(11), 372–379.

Patwardhan, B. and Mashelka, R.A. (2009). Traditional medicine inspired approaches to drug discovery: can Ayurveda show the way forward? *Drug Discov. Today* **14** (15–16), 804–811.

Pereira, D.M., Faria, J., Gaspar, L., Valentão, P., de Pinho, P.G. and Andrade, P.B. (2009). *Boerhaavia diffusa*: Metabolite profiling of a medicinal plant from Nyctaginaceae. *Food Chem. Toxicol.* **47**, 2142–2149.

Ponnusankar, S., Pandit, S., Babu, R., Bandyopadhyay, A. and Mukherjee, P.K. (2011a). Cytochrome P450 inhibitory potential of *Triphala* — a rasayana from Ayurveda. *J. Ethnopharmacol.* **133**, 120–125.

Ponnusankar, S., Pandit, S., Venkatesh, M., Bandyopadhyay, A. and Mukherjee, P.K. (2011b). Cytochrome P450 inhibition assay for standardized extract of *Terminalia chebula* Retz. *Phytother. Res.* **25**(1), 151–154.

Raskin, I., Ribnicky, D.M., Komarnytsky, S., Ilic, N., Poulev, A., Borisjuk, N., *et al.* (2002). Plants and human health in the twenty–first century. *Trends Biotechnol.* **20**, 522–531.

Sen, S., Chakraborty, R. and De, B. (2011). Challenges and opportunities in the advancement of herbal medicine: India's position and role in a global context. *J. Herb. Med.* **1**, 67–75.

Shirolkar, A., Gahlaut, A., Hooda, V. and Dabur, R. (2013). Phytochemical composition changes in untreated stem juice of *Tinospora cordifolia* (W) Mier during refrigerated storage. *J. Pharm. Res.* **7**, 1–6.

The Ayurvedic pharmacopoeia of India (2001). *Ministery of Health and Family Welfare, Department of ISM and H.* 1st Edition; Part I, Vol III, Government of India, New Delhi.

Trethewey, R. (2004). Metabolite profiling as an aid to metabolic engineering in plants. *Curr. Opin. Plant Biol.* **7**, 196–201.

WHO (2004). WHO bulletin: New alternative medicine guide launched amidst increasing reports of adverse reactions.

Zhang, L.W., Al-Suwayeh, S.A., Hsieh, P.W. and Fang, J.Y. (2010). A comparison of skin delivery of ferulic acid and its derivatives: evaluation of their efficacy and safety. *Int. J. Pharm.* **399**, 44–51.

Chapter 7

Natural Healing: *Qi Gong*, *Tai Chi* and Yoga

Ping-Chung Leung

Abstract

For thousands of years, a unique system of health promotion using natural means, *viz.* food, life style and exercises, has developed, matured and has been widely practised in China and India. "Natural Healing" might not be the best term to describe this system of health promotion but it is difficult to create more appropriate terminologies. One direct translation of this system of health promotion could be the maintenance or promotion of wellness. Natural Healing for Traditional Chinese Medicine (TCM) comprises the three components of physical, physiological and psychosocial harmony which are all interlinked. The ancient healers have worked out varieties of means to help bolstering the state of harmony.

Keywords: Natural Healing; *Qi Gong*; *Tai Chi*; Yoga; Stretching; Respiratory Control; Meditation.

7.1 Introduction

Natural Healing as a means to promote health and treating diseases is becoming popular in Europe and America. If Natural Healing refers to the maintenance of Health without specific drug or other means of treatment, it has long existed in China and India. For thousands of years, a unique system of health promotion using natural means, *viz.* food, life style and exercises, has developed, matured and has been widely practised in China and India. "Natural Healing" might not be the best term to describe this system of health promotion but it is difficult to create more appropriate terminologies. One direct translation of this system of health promotion could be the maintenance or promotion of wellness. Wellness refers to the physical, physiological, and psycho-social aspects of living through careful self-endeavours of food intake, life styles and exercises (Wang, 2008; Huang, 2009).

Joseph Needham pointed out in his great work on *History of Science and Technology in China* that the system of self-performed health maintenance in Ancient China never existed anywhere else in the world. Indeed, Natural Healing (we still use this terminology in view of the lack of appropriate substitute for a general understanding) in Chinese medicine exists as a complete system with a strong philosophical basis, involves careful conceptualisations, complicated methodologies of practice, and in recent years, commands organised social networks for its promotion (Wang, 2007; Lic, 2003). Ayurvedic medicine might not be as organised, but certainly is comparable to Chinese medicine in this area of wellness.

7.2 Philosophical Background

Natural Healing is strongly linked to the philosophy of Taoism. The philosopher Zuangtze used a colourful story to illustrate his thoughts about the clever utilisation of a tool which reflected to the living of one's life. An experienced butcher used his cutting knife for 19 years and found that it remained sharp. Of course, the butcher skilfully cut through the joints of the animals to get the meat out and never hit his knife against the hard bones. Human life could remain colourful and pleasant only if one could avoid the tough currents and be able to maintain the best performance.

Another Taoist, Laotze, stressed about the importance of "plainness and laxity", i.e. a state of utter mental relaxation away from worldly pursues, as a means to longevity. The Hindu Gods and Saints share the equivalent wisdoms.

Although Taoists probably have given the most solid input to the philosophical basis of Natural Healing in China, the system of health maintenance has been influenced by other philosophical schools. At the very beginning, spiritual dancing which was linked with superstitious spiritual worship to get rid of misfortunes, initiated certain forms of exercises which evolved through superstition to health purposes. Then when Confucians talked about celestial observations, meteorology, climate changes and their influences on human activities, health was brought to a level of interaction between the Human and Heavenly Divine. All these Taoist and Confucian inputs must be responsible for the meditation aspect of Natural Healing in China. Buddhism came to China from India later during the Tang period. Buddhists' practice of meditation with special requirements on the sitting posture then supplied additional influence in the development of Natural Healing (Ji, 1994a, 1994b).

7.3 Concepts of Natural Healing

One of the mostly emphasised areas of Health in the earliest classic of Chinese medicine, Ne-jing, is Natural Healing. Natural Healing — maintaining a perfect state of physical and physiological survival, as well as a harmonious state of psychosocial well-being, is considered the goal of Health and longevity.

The overall concept involves the harmony between *Yin* and *Yang*; harmony between physique and psychosocial state; balanced nutrition, balanced exercises and recreation. The concept of *Qi* is the most important for Natural Healing. When *Qi* remains healthy, abnormal physiological processes will not happen. *Qi* is the fundamental basis of survival, viability and vitality. *Qi* controls activities, changes and development. *Qi* has a direct form of respiration when air is inhaled through the nose to the lungs, thence, distributed throughout the body, along the meridians. *Qi* perpetuates on its own but needs continuous sustenance and reinforcement to maintain healthy development. Sustenance and reinforcement depends on repeated input of nutritional support and special exercises. *Qi* is not only the visible process of respiration which forms only the fundamental basis, *Pt* is also a state of physiological harmony expressed as perfect survival and good living. *Qi* is, at the same time, an inner feeling of internal balance, well-being and capability (Ji, 1994c, 1994d, 1994e).

Qi does not exist alone. *Qi* co-exists with two other special states which in modern terms, could be understood as a state of balanced secretion (精 *Jing*) and a state of spiritual esteem (神 *Shen*). Detailed physiology is not known to the ancient healers, but they have good knowledge about visible secretions like saliva and secretions from the bowel and genitals. Their concept of "secretion" in fact has combined the exocrine and endocrine systems. Therefore, *Jing* could be understood as a fundamental state of exocrine and endocrine balance. The state of spiritual esteem is easily interpreted today as psychosocial well-being (Si, 2006; Liang, 2005).

Natural Healing for Traditional Chinese Medicine (TCM), therefore, comprises the three components of physical, physiological and psychosocial harmony which are all interlinked. The ancient healers, through so many years of practice, have worked out varieties of means to help bolstering the state of harmony.

7.4 Practice of Natural Healing

When Natural Healing is discussed, either under the popular European or American concept of today, or is considered with a modern Chinese medicine context, it is commonly taken as activities related with treatment of a straight forward disease entity or activities arranged for rehabilitation. In reality, Natural Healing in Chinese medicine has a much broader concept, which covers maintenance of health, wellness and prevention of falling sick.

The two best-known varieties of Natural Healing today are *Qi Gong* and *Tai Chi*; the former allows a lot of practitioner's modifications while the latter follows a rigid system of chained activities (Yi, 2007; Wang and Xiang, 2006).

Qi Gong

The promotion of Natural Healing requires disciplined practices that would help bringing harmony to the three important components, *viz. Jing*, *Shen* and *Qi*.

Stretching

Historically, spiritual dancing could have been the very early practice of Natural Healing. Hence, stretching movements while adopting a variety of postures have become the most essential components of practice. Early imitation of the postures of different animals have later evolved into chains of movements copying animal activities. Later, still different groups of practitioners created their own system of activities and motions with different connotations and hallmarks. The uniform component of these different systems is that all of them consist of stretching movements. As far as posture is concerned some advocate natural postures like standing, sitting; modifications like "Buddha sitting", half-kneeling, animal postures, etc.

Respiratory Control

The practice of Natural Healing invariably included controlled breathing without which there will be little value of the stretching exercises. *Qi Gong* might have inaccurately been assumed that it deals with *Qi* only. In fact, it is the sustenance and development of the *Qi* that requires simultaneous stretching, controlled respiration and meditation. It is believed that with skilful control of breathing, *Qi* is manipulated successfully, so that it not only circulates through the respiratory system, but together with meditation, it reaches the different physiological systems to improve their metabolic state of balance.

Respiration is controlled so that the normal pattern is not followed. The recommended patterns include extra-long inspiration or extra-long expiration while the latter is preferred. Abdominal or diaphragmatic breathing is also practised. While doing so, the pelvic diaphragm and anal sphincters are also squeezed at will.

So, respiratory control is executed simultaneously with the stretching movements in a smooth synchronised chain of activities under the individual's free will. It would be up to the individual to develop his/her own policy of training which could be amended from time to time (Yang, 2001; Won, 2004).

Meditation

Natural Healing aims at harmonising physical, humoral and mental activities. Meditation is an indispensable component. The intersectional harmony must be promoted. The skilful practitioner attains a tranquillity of the mind while stretching is being performed with controlled breathing. It must be understood that meditation requires the simultaneous support from stretching and breathing and *vice versa*. The apparently complicated system of movements in *Tai Chi* should not be hindering meditation. Rather, they provide a good initiating environment where the day-to-day mental pressure will not be felt. The material background for meditation is resting of the central nervous system. During the training, the intention is to give a good rest to the central nervous system: free it from motor and sensory burdens, (apart from the comforting limb movements) relieve it from complex memories, protect it from emotions and problem solving requirements. The assumption is that with this unchallenged mental state, a reorganisation of the interacting neurological messages can take place, initiating a neurological establishment of harmony and a reorganised humoral state (Won, 2008; Chen, 1998).

Tai Chi

While all the three components (stretching, controlled breathing and meditation) are stressed and must be practised in the training, different schools of promotion keen to initiate modifications would find the stretching part most versatile for change. *Tai Chi*, for instance, allows colourful dancing movements with varying speeds. The whole set of arrangements is established after thorough consideration of the meridians and sites of the acupoints.

Tai Chi requires a fully relaxed body. While the four limbs moves in semicircular and circular movements, the focus remains around the waist, which rotates left and right. The movements stimulate the 300 acupoints of the whole body in a orchestrated manner. The result is a concerted, systematic stimulation of the acupoints, each one of which is related to certain somatic or sympathetic functions. All *Tai Chi* practitioners are aware of the circulatory activations once the *Tai Chi* exercises continue for a while. Recent functional magnetic resonance investigation on brain function also has preliminary evidences to show that the stimulation of acupuncture points does elicit functional changes in different parts of the brain (Jones, 2001; Hsu, 1986).

In fact, the term *Tai Chi* is self-explanatory. Just imagine the *Tai Chi* symbol which is a round circular figure within which harbours two fish symbols, that go along a clockwise chase after each other (see Symbol of *Tai Chi*). *Tai Chi*, therefore, signifies the natural law of the universe, which is possessing perfect harmony and balance. Followers should therefore obey the law of balance between light and heavy, slow and fast, weak and strong, keep a well-controlled breathing, avoid jerky motions, over strenuous movements, etc. Movements of the left and right arms could be viewed as *Yin* and *Yang* forces. The aim is to maintain their balance. Every movement in *Tai Chi* needs to be synchronised with respiration. The concerted contractions of the muscle groups require gentle oxygen intake and then join together and converge into a state of *Qi* establishment (Green and Blankshy, 1996; Chang and Wai, 1997).

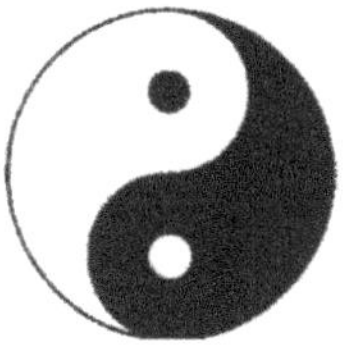

Symbol of *Tai Chi* 太極圖

Students practising *Qi Gong* and *Tai Chi* are advised to be aware of four states of mind during the exercises:

(i) *A sense of central stability*: *Qi Gong* principle states that *Qi* starts with the nose, follows the midline trachea to the lungs, thence, follows the central line anteriorly along the midline to the umbilical region and at the central back to the upper lumbar region. Limb movements and body rotation are centred along this central pillar of *Qi*. With this concept in mind, *Tai Chi* performance is relaxed and accurate (Motoyama and sunami, 1998).

According to *Tai Chi* trainers, poor performances are related to a lack of understanding of controlled breathing, ignorance about training regulations, about the timing of adding strength, and failure to master the concept of *Yin–Yang* balance. Moreover, *Tai Chi* practice should not be overenergetic, otherwise, the pressure of quick achievement would affect relaxation and the need for meditation (Astsumi, 2007).

(ii) *Awareness of the bony prominence*: Bony prominences are all related to muscle attachments. Like the acupoints along the meridians, *Tai Chi* movements give them indirect stimulations. Intentional stretching relevant to the bony prominences have additional stimulation effects.

(iii) *State of awareness relevant to the meridians*: The practising person should have a sound knowledge about the meridians and bear in mind the position of the acupoints during practice so that with a certain posture and a special movement, appropriate stimulation can be given to the relevant acupoints.

(iv) *State of tranquillity*: After sufficient time of practice, *Tai Chi* gives the practitioner not only the usual relaxed state of calm and pleasure, but a an additional feeling of unworldliness, sometimes described as the state of euphoria experienced by a half-drunken individual. This pleasant state has been considered a measurement of achievement.

7.5 Clinical Research on *Qi Gong* and *Tai Chi*

Epidemiological surveys on people enjoying long life all showed that the common components for longevity include very good quality of life ever since they are born. Thus, the Okinawa study on centurions showed that these people living beyond 100 years had balanced healthy diet, plenty of exercise and rich healthy social activities (Astsumi, 2007).

People practising *Qi Gong* and *Tai Chi* realise that through gentle, disciplined exercises, they gain sustained muscular strength, general vitality and mental tranquillity. They have reasons to believe that they become healthier and would live longer. People practising *Tai Chi* and *Qi Gong* also claim that they do not fall sick and are not vulnerable to diseases. Those might be simple evidences supporting the Chinese Way of Natural Healing as being good for the prevention of diseases.

With the rising popularity of Natural Healing and the oriental influence on the perception of health, more and more people have started to practice *Qi Gong* and *Tai Chi*. Academics and professionals have started to seriously look for the scientific basis of the Chinese Way of Natural Healing. Many reports on the clinical effects of *Qi Gong* and *Tai Chi* have appeared in the past decade. The following paragraphs attempt to give a glimpse of the research being done.

Qi Gong

In 2004, the Beijing Sport University conducted a clinical study on the effects of *Qi Gong* on the physical ability of a group of people aged from 50 to 70. Fifteen days of *Qi Gong* exercises were given to these people, after which their physical fitness was assessed and compared with their pre-study conditions. Parameters of assessment included basic musculoskeletal data like body weight, waist girdle, fat thickness, hand grip strength, leg strength and stance. Heart–lung fitness was also measured. The results showed that the basic physical state of the people under training, i.e. body weight, girdle and fat thickness, etc. did not change. The musculoskeletal activities, as were manifested by hand grip and leg strength, improved. Balancing power also significantly improved. With regard to cardio-pulmonary health. The heart rate showed a steady state before and after the training period. Looking at the heart rate changes during the *Qi Gong* exercise, it was shown that the maximal, median and finishing heart rates all improved (lowered) towards the end of the training. This is a clear indication that the ability of the heart among this group of middle age and older age people to adapt to higher demand of physical activities improved with the *Qi Gong*. Respiratory function also improved after the period of training (Tsang and Chow, 2005).

In 2005, the Sports Institute of the Jiangxi University conducted a study on the cardiac function of 70 people, aged between 61 and 68, in response to a continuous training of *Qi Gong* of Stretching. The training lasted six months. A control group of 30 people was recruited, having quite similar body weights and heights. Cardiac function was assessed using high resolution ultrasonic equipment. The chosen parameters included stroke volume (SV), early diastolic velocity (VE) and late diastolic velocity (VA).

Table 7.1. Cardiac function before and after training.

	Control group ($n = 31$)		Study group ($n = 39$)	
	Before training	After six months' training	Before training	After six months' training
SV (mL)	57.94 ± 16.01	58.51 ± 16.99	55.72 ± 15.78	67.15 ± 13.67**#
VE (cm/s)	65.95 ± 19.95	66.30 ± 19.75	66.50 ± 18.24	75.05 ± 17.66**#
VA (cm/s)	84.36 ± 15.12	82.68 ± 14.10	83.02 ± 13.89	83.76 ± 15.21
VE–VA	−18.41 ± 23.98	−16.38 ± 24.68	−16.53 ± 25.96	−10.25 ± 23.32*

The results in Table 7.1. showed better SV and VE in the trained group compared with the control group. VE–VA showed even a more convincing improvement (Du *et al.*, 2006).

On a related theme of cardiovascular function, changes in the serum fatty acid levels were studied before and after *Qi Gong* in the Talien Institute of Physical Training in 2008. For this study, 62 patients with high serum triglyceride levels were selected and randomly divided into the trial and control groups. The trial group was instructed for training on a scheme of 60 minutes per day for six months. Parameters of assessment included the molecular markers S1 CAM-1, SVCAM-1, Ps, Fig, TG, TC, LDL-C and HDL-C levels. After six months of *Qi Gong* exercises, HDL-C was higher in the study group while all the other markers were lower than the control group (Yen, 2009; Brevetti and Schiano, 2006).

The effects of different types of Guang'anmen diabetes patients have been studied. The Beijing Guang-on-mun Hospital, in collaboration with Japanese clinicians, conducted a clinical study on 108 type 2 diabetic patients, divided into four different groups: Group 1 practised stretching *Qi Gong*; Group 2 practised static *Qi Gong* (without stretching); Group 3 practised both stretching and static *Qi Gong* and Group 4 was the control, not practising *Qi Gong*. Observations lasted four months. Parameters included fasting blood sugar, and quality of Life (QoL) indices. Assessments were done before training, two and four months after training. The best results were observed in Group 3 where all parameters, including objective blood tests and QoL improved after four months' training and the results were better than the control group.

Results of the Groups 1 and 2 also showed similar but less impressive trends (Lin and Wang, 2009).

In 2002, psychologists in Jiangxi conducted a research on the cognitive state and mental ability of elderly people aged 50–70, before and after six months' *Qi Gong* training. The assessment tool used was a software invented by Suen *et al.* in 1989, which tested the mental speed taken to solve simple mathematical problems, identification of symbols and sketches, motor reactions, memory, and imitations. It was shown that the haemoglobin A1 and mental ability of the *Qi Gong* group improved significantly compared with the untrained group (Chang *et al.*, 2006; Suen *et al.*, 1989).

For all musculoskeletal training, motor improvement could mean positive effects on the bones as well. The Shantung Technical University has conducted a research on 60 people with known osteoporosis in 2008. The study group practised *Qi Gong* daily for a period of 60 minutes, assessment included pain symptoms on an analogue scale, bone mineral density measurement, serum alkaline phosphatase and other bone metabolism parameters. The end results after training (exact duration not given) showed significant improvement in bone health and bone mineral density.

Tai Chi

It might seem beyond anybody's doubt that *Tai Chi* exercises will have general as well as musculoskeletal effects on those who diligently practice it. The impression could be that it is particularly suitable for the elderly people. *Tai Chi* is certainly more popular than *Qi Gong*, although the three components — stretching, controlled breathing and meditation — are common to both. The dancing movements of *Tai Chi* could be the real motivating force for beginners.

Studies have shown that not only would disease-free people find benefits with the *Tai Chi* training, but also those suffering from musculoskeletal weaknesses, e.g. after chronic work-related back injuries could rely on *Tai Chi* exercises either as a solitary form of treatment, or as adjuvant therapy. One well-designed study was completed in two hospitals in Shanxi. Sixty four patients suffering from work-related spinal degeneration unrelated to other organic pathology were divided into two groups at

Table 7.2. Treatment results in 4, 8, 12 week.

Group	Number	Male/ Female	Recovered	Improved	No improvement	Cure rate	Effectiveness (%)
4 weeks							
Control	32	20/12	2	27	3	6.3	90.6
Tai Chi	32	22/10	4	28	1	9.4	96.9
8 weeks							
Control	32	20/12	40	21	1	31.3	96.9
Tai Chi	32	22/10	18	14	0	56.3*	100
12 weeks							
Control	32	20/12	22	10	0	68.8	100
Tai Chi	32	22/10	27	5	0	84.4**	100

*$p < 0.01$; ** $p < 0.05$.

random. One group was instructed to use *Tai Chi* as training, the other group received massage and physiotherapy. Results of treatment indicated positive benefits with *Tai Chi* at different stages of treatment (Chen, 2009; Shao and Zhou, 2008) (Table 7.2).

Tai Chi should be particularly good for training muscle balance in the lower limbs. A large scale comparative study was done in Beijing, covering 421 people on regular *Tai Chi* practice and others not doing sports. The study aimed at revealing whether *Tai Chi* would improve balancing power. A single test of one leg stand with blinded vision was used. The durations of stance was taken as objective data. Results showed uniform improvement in the *Tai Chi* group.

In this study, the method of assessing balance appeared too crude, and the differences between training and without training could be repeated using other assessment methodology (Taggart *et al.*, 2003; Maki, 1990). Like *Qi Gong*, *Tai Chi* is known to have cardio-pulmonary supporting effects on the trainees. A study was conducted in Fujian on 39 middle aged and elderly people before and after they started training, which lasted one year. Using the cardiac function monitor, the following data were collected: stroke volume (SV), stroke index (SI), Cardiac output (CO), pulse rate (PR), heart oxygen consumption volume (HOV) and

Table 7.3. Changes in cardiac function.

Indices	1996	1997	Rate
PR (min)	76.18 ± 11.73	72.08 ± 9.18**	5.38
SV (mL)	81.14 ± 1.72	84.05 ± 16.86*	3.59
CO (L/min)	6.10 ± 1.05	6.42 ± 1.20*	5.29
SI (mL/m^2)	53.15 ± 9.51	55.41 ± 7.52*	4.24
HOI	2629.74 ± 616.08	2517.58 ± 593.45*	4.27
HOV (mL/min)	43.82 ± 10.27	40.23 ± 6.94*	8.19

*$p < 0.05$, **$p < 0.01$.

heart oxygen consumption index (HOI). The results are summarised in (Table 7.3) (Lui *et al.*, 2001).

If *Tai Chi* is good for cardiac health, what about its effect on hypertension? The general mediating effects of exercises on hypertensive individuals are well accepted. Researchers from Sichuan have done a study on 124 patients suffering from essential hypertension, encouraging them to do *Tai Chi* exercises or therapeutic walking as means to help the standard drug treatment. Both groups showed positive effects with exercises, but the *Tai Chi* group did better. Patients with milder increases in blood pressure also did better than those with severe hypertension (Wang *et al.*, 2007; Mao, 2002; Wang, 2002).

Since *Tai Chi* helps with hypertension, one could assume that the complex system of stretching, controlled breathing and meditation, has humoral effects like controlling serum fatty acids and immunological influences. Public health experts in Sichuan University studied 72 *Tai Chi* exercisers and 55 controls to look at their serum antioxidants, *viz.* superoxide dismutase (SOD), glutathione peroxidase (GSH-Px), catalase (CAT) and malondialdehyde (MDA). Results showed that SOD, GSH-Px and CAT functions in the control group were higher than the *Tai Chi* group ($p < 0.05$) while MDA was lower ($p < 0.05$). Looking at the differences between the exercises of different durations, it is interesting to note that the longer the practice and experience, the more active were the antioxidants (Table 7.4) (Huang *et al.*, 2001; Tao and Tung, 1988).

Groups of gerontologists observed in recent years that deteriorating health and decline of physical performance of elderly people are often

Table 7.4. Relationship between different duration of *Tai Chi* practice.

	1–5 years		5–10 years		Over 10 years	
Markers	*n*	$x \pm s$	*n*	$x \pm s$	*n*	$x \pm s$
SOD (NU/mL)	37	78.28 ± 15.27	21	99.66 ± 13.16	13	104.1 ± 12.48
GSH-Px (U/mL)	36	58.08 ± 2.88	22	72.21 ± 11.52	13	77.79 ± 8.75
CA T (U/mL)	37	1.78 ± 0.20	21	2.02 ± 0.19	13	2.05 ± 0.14
MDA (nmol/mL)	29	4.54 ± 0.19	10	4.03 ± 0.39	8	3.62 ± 0.17

Note: Differences all reaching $p < 0.05$.

related to subclinical deficiencies of endocrine functions, particularly of the thyroid gland and gonads. Sports scientists in Shanghai investigated 51 elderly *Tai Chi* exercisers (60–90 years), comparing them with 47 elderly (60–80 years) and 17 young adults (24–50 years). Serum markers included testosterone (T), estrogen (E2), luteohormone (LH), follicular stimulating hormone (FSH), thyroid stimulating hormone (TSH), thyroxin 4 (T4) and prolactin (PRL). Table 7.5 shows the interesting results, indicating decline in the hormone levels, with age. However, *Tai Chi* helps to alleviate some of the deficiencies (Hsu and Wang, 1986).

Table 7.5. Differences in serum hormone level.

Serum hormone level	*Tai Chi* group	Elderly group	Young group	P		
				A:B	B:C	A:C
F (ng/dL)	14.74 ± 4.73	15.23 ± 7.67	14.20 ± 3.92	> 0.05	> 0.05	> 0.05
TSH (μU/mL)	4.80 ± 3.05	3.80 ± 1.55	3.10 ± 1.15	< 0.05	> 0.05	< 0.05
T_3 (ng/mL)	0.93 ± 0.20	0.84 ± 0.21	1.51 ± 0.31	< 0.05	< 0.01	< 0.05
T_4 (ng/mL)	69.97 ± 23.87	73.60 ± 31.96	104.97 ± 38.60	> 0.05	< 0.05	< 0.01
$_rT_3$ (ng/mL)	30.26 ± 7.77	28.79 ± 4.96	37.22 ± 7.64	> 0.05	< 0.01	< 0.01
FSH (mIU/mL)	16.54 ± 15.16	11.05 ± 6.08	4.85 ± 1.58	< 0.05	< 0.01	< 0.01
LH (mIU/mL)	11.74 ± 13.19	8.03 ± 5.95	4.41 ± 1.31	> 0.05	< 0.01	< 0.05
T (ng/dL)	680.00 ± 430.00*	510.00 ± 151.00	679.00 ± 173.00**	< 0.05	< 0.01	> 0.05
E_2 (pg/mL)	63.91 ± 17.14	54.74 ± 18.62$^{\Delta}$	50.70 ± 7.14$^{\Delta\Delta}$	< 0.05	> 0.05	< 0.05
PRL (ng/mL)	7.06 ± 3.46	6.34 ± 2.75	8.25 ± 3.21	> 0.05	> 0.05	> 0.05

*$n = 50$; ** $n = 12$; $^{\Delta}n = 46$; $^{\Delta\Delta}n = 10$.

Like Qi Gong, *Tai Chi* is believed to have preventive function against infection and other pathological changes. Investigating immunology related changes should throw light on the assumption. The interleukins (IL's) are a group of cytokines created by mononuclear cells regulating cellular activities. IL2 is probably the most important member which controls the survival of T cells, NK cells and B cells, and is actively involved in anti-cancer activities.

Scholars in the College of Martial Arts, Beijing, have carried out a study to investigate the interleukin changes in 16 health women, aged between 55 and 65. Ten were *Tai Chi* exercisers while 6 were controls. After six months of exercises, the exercise group, which already had higher concentration of IL2, showed further increases. For those who already finished six months of *Tai Chi* training, even one single round of *Tai Chi* exercises, lasting one hour, boosted up the IL2 level to a statistically significant degree (from 100.3 ± 20.46 to 110.7 ± 20, $p < 0.01$) (Wang, 2003; Lewicki, 1988).

One of the intended effects of *Tai Chi* is a state of psychological balance like *Qi Gong*. Some studies have been designed to look at the contribution of *Tai Chi* on the psychological state of exercisers. Hundred and thirty three elderly people were recruited in Xian. They were divided into three groups: *Tai Chi* practice, free exercisers, and control group with no exercises.

Their psychological states were assessed at zero, two and six months, using the Cornell University Mental Assessment index (CMA). With this assessment index, psychological explorations included symptoms of depression, anxiety and tension. Included in the questionnaire were also symptoms of the vital systems: respiratory, cardiovascular, gastrointestinal, muscular-skeletal, neurological, etc. Frequency of fatigue and illnesses was also explored. The results of the study showed a general improvement on the psychological parameters, reaching statistical significance, while the other functional indices are also shown to the advantage of the *Tai Chi* group (Yi, 2008).

7.6 Effects of Yoga and *Qi Gong* Practice on Mental Health

In the first place, both systems of physical training aim at the attainment of meditation i.e. mental serenity as the terminal stage of the self-disciplined exercises. Reaching the meditation level requires repeated practices and is subjectively felt by the individual. In the past decade, Magnetic Resonance Studies carried out in different institutes have demonstrated that functional activities in different regions of the brain could be affected by sustained postures, musculoskeletal stretches and controlled breathings. These observations are early objective indications of the neurological outcome of Yoga and *Qi Gong* (Kirkwood *et al.*, 2005).

With the complexity of Neuro-Anatomy and Neuro-Physiology, it might take decades to get nearer to the scientific depths of how Yoga or *Qi Gong* influences brain functions. At this stage, we only have clinical evidences from different parts of the world, about the clinical values of Yoga and *Qi Gong* on the maintenance of mental health, from prevention to treatment of anxiety disorders and depression.

Yoga

In 2005, a systematic review on the effects of Yoga on anxiety was completed in the University of Westminister, United Kingdom. Eight studies were reviewed. In spite of many inadequacies in the methodologies, it appeared that many cases of anxiety state benefited from Yoga, although specific recommendations could not be made (45).

The same group reviewed the effects of Yoga for depression in 2005. They analysed five randomised controlled trials which all reported positive results although the study methodologies were not perfect (Pilkington *et al.*, 2005).

A systematic review done in Australia in 2008 on the effectiveness of Yoga and self-help for anxiety disorders found that Yoga was superior to medications like diazepam (Penman *et al.*, 2012).

Looking through many other reviews of different academic levels, one realises the general trend of encouraging results, which has been summarised in Table 7.6.

Many other solitary reports on the effects of Yoga on the Mental State of people suffering from different degrees of anxiety disorders are available. Exercise training alone has been proven clinically effective in major depression and panic disorders (Khalsa, 2004). Yoga should also provide enhancing effects on standard treatments. Since those maintained on antipsychotic medications are more vulnerable to obesity, diabetes and heart diseases, Yoga would be particularly indicated (Harvard Mental Health

Table 7.6. Yoga and meditation for stress, anxiety, anxiety disorders mood disorders, sleep disorders and depression.

Source of study	Summary of results
Arias *et al.* (2006) systematic review USA	82 studies, 20 RCTs. The strongest evidence for efficacy was found for epilepsy, symptoms of premenstrual syndrome and menopausal symptoms. Benefit was also demonstrated for non-psychotic mood and anxiety disorders, autoimmune illness and emotional disturbance in neoplastic disease.
Krisanaprakornkit *et al.* (2006) systematic review Thailand	Only two studies eligible for inclusion. Anti-anxiety drugs were continued in both. The duration of trials ranged from 12 to 18 weeks. Transcendental Meditation showed a reduction in anxiety symptoms.
Lafferty *et al.* (2006) systematic review USA	27 clinical trials investigating massage or mind–body interventions, 26 showed significant improvements in symptoms such an anxiety, emotional distress, comfort, nausea and pain, difficult to judge the clinical significance of the results.
Kirkwood *et al.* (2005) systematic review UK	Eight studies all reported positive results, quality of studies was poor and no firm conclusions can be drawn.
Pilkington *et al.* (2005) systematic review UK	Five RCTs found that overall, yoga interventions for depressive disorders were potentially beneficial; however, methodological limitations prevented drawing firm conclusions.
Astin *et al.* (2003) systematic review USA	There were moderate evidence of efficacy for mind-body therapies in the areas of hypertension and arthritis.
Jorm *et al.* (2004) review Australia	Review for anxiety disorders found the treatments with the best evidence of effectiveness were kava, exercise, relaxation training and bibliotherapy.

letter, 2009; Brown and Gerbarg, 2005a), especially for those who are not suitable for aerobic exercises.

Since the 1970's, meditation and other stress-reduction techniques are more and more frequently practised and studied as possible means of treatments for depression and anxiety. The practice of Yoga, which combines exercises with meditation, unfortunately has been under-looked. The Harvard Medical School Health Review reported that in the recent decades an increasing number of Yoga practices revealed that Yoga reduced the unfavourable influences of exaggerated stress responses, hence should be helpful for anxiety and depression, equivalent to other self-soothing techniques like therapeutic relaxation, meditation and socialisation. Yoga also helped through easing respiration and reducing heart rate which were considered indicators of the bodily ability to response to stress (Brown and Gerbarg, 2005b). The tolerability to pain was also increased. Another study at Harvard found that at the end of three months, women in a Yoga group reported improvements in perceived stress, depression, anxiety, energy, fatigue and well-being. Depression scores improved by 50%, anxiety scores by 30% and overall well-being by 65%. Initial complaints of headaches, back pain and poor sleep quality also resolved much more often in the Yoga group than in the control group (Janakiramaiah *et al.*, 2000).

A review on Yoga would not be qualified without screening reports from India herself. Indeed, the majority of research on Yoga has been conducted by Indian investigators and published in Indian journals, although there are increasing contributors from US and England, and increasing applications of Yoga are included in the new specialty of mind–body medicine (Khalsa, 2004). A study done in Bangalore India in 2000, comparing the antidepressant effects between Yoga, medication with imipramine, and electro-convulsive therapy for melancholia, showed that significant reductions in the total score rating of depression occurred in all three groups. At week 3, the Yoga group scored higher than the electro-convulsive group but was not different from the medication group. Remission rates at the end of the trial were 93%, 73% and 67% in the electro-convulsive, medication and Yoga groups, respectively (Janakiramaiah *et al.*, 2000).

Qi Gong

As stated earlier, *Qi Gong* is composed mainly of three essential self-attained activities, *viz.* stretching across joints, controlled breathing and meditation. Which mechanisms are most important towards the accomplishment of a physiological harmony presenting as both physical and mental well-being? Many theories have been postulated. One theory emphasises on muscle relaxation, claiming that relaxation brings about improved blood circulation, better oxygen provision and removal of metabolic wastes. Another theory and limited experiments have shown the enhancement of the immunological defence. It is observed that relaxation, and controlled breathing could be giving the mind an effective training to relieve stress and pain. Other scientists have demonstrated changing hormonal levels in the blood during *Qi Gong* practice, while at the same time suppressing sympathetic output (Shi *et al.*, 2005; Shi, 2005).

With regard to research publications on *Qi Gong*, plentiful are available in Chinese language journals but the methodologies of studies are largely of low quality. The reports are mostly from sports related studies and analyses tend to be superficial.

A report from Wuhan, China, on the elderlies practising *Qi Gong* showed that six weeks' practice reduced anxiety and depression primarily felt by the individuals while cardiac and pulmonary functions also improved (Shi *et al.*, 2005). Another study completed in Shanxi in 2005 approached from the ancient Chinese philosophers' context, but whether Confucian or Taoist philosophical views are suitable for the interpretation of harmonising observations remain controversial (Shi, 2005).

A controlled study was done in 2006 on 600 people practising and not practising *Qi Gong*. Those who had long experience were found to have more stable mental health (Zhai, 2006).

A group of hospital workers in USA were given *Qi Gong* training for six weeks after which they were assessed using the Perceived Stress Scale together with the quality of life, questionnaire, using the SF36 questionnaire. The outcome was compared with another group of hospital workers not trained. The *Qi Gong* group demonstrated statistically significant reduction of perceived stress compared to the control group ($p = 0.02$) Greater improvement on the quality of life was also found in the *Qi Gong* group (Griffith *et al.*, 2008).

Medical Students who practised *Qi Gong* for 12 weeks were studied on their mental adaptability including depression, anxiety, aggressiveness, threat, stubbornness and social behaviours. Hundred of them were compared with 50 others who did not practice *Qi Gong*. The practising group showed significantly higher scores ($p < 0.01$) (Liu *et al.*, 2008).

A detailed case study done in Sweden on the mood recovery of a woman who lost her job and became dreadfully distressed was most interesting. After practising *Qi Gong*, the woman was found to be continuously benefit from the exercises. Exercise behaviour was recorded daily, stress-energy and wellness were followed up weekly and mindfulness after 4, 9 and 12 weeks. The woman felt that her mental state was enjoying progressive stabilisation to high levels: she could better adapt to stressful situations and was less worried about unexpected mishap in life (Jouper and Johansson, 2013). She believed firmly that *Qi Gong* was the main cause of her mental improvements.

Reports about mental health after Yoga and *Qi Gong* training on the whole, are giving rather vague ideas of the state of the mind. "Stable mental health" is often stated. To the experts on mental health and psychiatrists, it might mean little because specific psychiatric symptoms are not described.

7.7 Discussions

We have briefly reviewed the history of Natural Healing in China, its philosophical background, conceptualisation within the practice of Chinese Medicine, similarities with Indian Medicine, the procedural requirements, claims and recent scientific endeavours to reveal the physiological basis of the two most popular exercises, *viz. Qi Gong* and *Tai Chi*. It would be appropriate to give more general discussions, and to approach more from the common sense aspect so as to try answering one question — "Should I practice *Qi Gong* or *Tai Chi* or Yoga?"

Natural Healing in Europe and US might have specific demands and needs. Natural Healing in the oriental sense is more of a promotion of wellness and longevity, although those people threatened by diseases or ill-health might have their special needs and demands. We might not feel particularly threatened by the imagination of a special disease, but we certainly do not want to fall sick. We might not particularly adore and work for longevity, but again, we do not want to fall sick. If not falling sick could be achieved through the simple procedures of stretching exercises, controlled breathing and meditation, it would certainly be most inviting. If the tripartite procedures can be easily learned, comfortably practised and more importantly, freely modified, they would earn even greater popularity and deserve more promotions.

Looking at the modifications of the procedures involved in the exercises throughout the long period of its history, we could be quite confident about the flexibility that could be allowed. Since stretching exercises with different postures have been practised and recorded since over 3,000 years ago, countless numbers of practice system have evolved, bearing the same principles. All those systems of exercises, labelled with unique names of their own, have enjoyed genuine popularities and substantial groups of followers. When instructors take up the role of training new students, they naturally have a tendency to modify again the details. After all, not a single individual could claim the ability to exactly perform a muscular (motor) action that exactly matched another person's performance. Modification and diversion is therefore mandatory. After so many decades of intentional and unintentional modifications, exercises like *Qi Gong* and *Tai Chi* have retained their Natural Healing values. Individual modifications, as long as they are conforming to the basic concepts and requirements, should be allowed, even encouraged. Although different groups have rather rigid directions and contents of training and followers are instructed to closely follow, when they fail to do so perfectly, they are allowed to modify along their own abilities. If the system of exercises could be so freely modified, does it mean that individuals could just be acquainted with the procedures, adhere to the basic principles, and then creatively practice on their own?

I realise that different groups in China, on their own pursuing of Natural Healing, have already done that. The evidence could be found in the public parks in China today. Early in the morning in these parks, one finds people practising conventional *Qi Gong* and *Tai Chi*. One finds also other groups practising other innovative forms of stretching exercises which they have invented. One sees them engaged in modified folk dancing, social dancing, different stretches, etc. There are also those who walk with their backs leading the way. These are all innovative inventions of exercises basing on the principle of stretching.

What about the other area of controlled breathing? There are groups of people practising singing, or Peking opera. Others shout and/or yell in their own way of control, making colourful innovative varieties of controlled breathing. A few quietly Buddha-sit below the trees and are engaged in either conventional or their own way of controlled respiration. *Qi Gong* instructions have listed a variety of breathing patterns with short or long lengths at different stages of the breathing cycle and to be performed with different forces, through the chest cage or abdominal diaphragm. The varieties of advocated breathing patterns, in fact, have indirectly endorsed the feasibility of individualised innovative practices and have apparently encouraged the practices of singing and yelling.

Our current attitude could be the practice of stretching and controlled breathing, which after all promotes physical and psychological well-being that aspires to a superb tranquillity of the mind, and could be recommended to all. In fact, it could be a happy coincidence that the same requirements, *viz.* stretching, controlled breathing and meditation, are required in the popular Health Promotion exercise in India: the Yoga practice.

While the practice of Natural Healing in the Chinese Community is historical and cultural, it is also very personal. It is a personal habit that the individual has chosen to adopt. In a way, it resembles the eating habit and the sleeping habit that do not need any justification. Still, the individual could review it with the intension of modification or enforcement for one's own good. Scientific proof for the practice of *Qi Gong* and *Tai Chi* on one's well-being would not be required. However, nowadays, even well-being — wellness, could be physiologically or clinically defined and objective parameters are created for the measurement of wellness. Those who are converted to thorough, strict scientific explorations have started investigating the "objective value" of *Qi Gong*, *Tai Chi* and other Natural Healing practices.

I have already given examples of proper research studies reported from different institutions in China. From those reports, scattered evidences of favourable changes in various physiological areas have been shown. In fact, the interest on the Chinese way of Natural Healing has turned international. Japanese scholars have reported widely on the cardio-pulmonary effects of *Qi Gong* and *Tai Chi*, as well as their immunomodulating influences (Li and Chu, 2008; Chen and Chung, 2002). Likewise, the most influential research institution on health, NIH, USA, has many times encouraged research commitment on *Qi Gong* and *Tai Chi*. A recent report from NIH about a randomised controlled trial of 112 subjects aged 59–86 on *Tai Chi* exercises, against health education, using chicken pox vaccine as a stimulant to immunological responses, indicated that the *Tai Chi* group enjoyed a 40% increase in their immunological responses (double to that of the controls), and an improved physical and mental state of health (Whelton, 2002).

Let us go back to the basic question of "Should I practice *Qi Gong* or *Tai Chi* or Yoga?"

The popularity is clear. The popularity is historically and culturally linked. The practice requires little cost. The practice can be easily verified at different levels of personal practice.

But if one considers that scientific proof is of paramount importance, what we are clear today remains scanty, non-specific, and partial.

May be there is a hidden concept that could be revealed through careful observations on the practice of *Qi Gong* and *Tai Chi* and Yoga, particularly its procedures of stretching, controlled breathing and meditation.

What does stretching do? Stretching produces tension on the muscles, tendons, ligaments and the components of the joints. Stretching with chosen positions produces tension on some muscles, tendons, ligaments and joints that are normally not for active use. The Gate theory in neurophysiology confers that with every stretch and stimulation of the proprioceptive nerve receptor in the tendons and ligaments, messages are sent up to the brain to block up pain sensation and initiate other chains of events in the central nervous system. With every intentional stretch additional proprioceptive messages are sent up. When people walk backwards with their backs leading the way, what are happening? Muscle groups that are not normally active in walking are activated and they send out massive unusual proprioceptive messages to the brain.

What does controlled breathing do? Controlled breathing creates an unusual muscular (motor) system of events for respiratory function which follows a new sequence and pattern. The modified rates, intensities of inspiration and expiration, the different groups of muscles mobilised, together composed a totally novel, inexperienced system of motor activity. Stimulations received through these complex motor activities are new to the central nervous system. The stimulation is not only confined to the accustomed somatosensory system of neurological control. The respiratory control is mastered through both the somatic motor system, which allows voluntary control, and the autonomic (parasympathetic) nervous system, which is responsible for the automatic regulatory control of respiration. Intentional controlled breathing therefore is making use of the somatic nervous activity to initiate stimulations on the autonomic nervous system, which has wide connections with the internal organs. Controlled breathing therefore opens up new channels of communication with the internal organs under conscious intension. These new channels of communication, could give an explanation to the old concept of *Qi Gong* and *Tai Chi*, that the practice pushes the *Qi* through the internal organs to help building a state of physiological harmony.

What does meditation do? No one is free from the somatic stimulations and psychological disturbances that bother him endlessly. One does enjoy a good rest during night time sleep. Unfortunately, with overload of accumulative worldly events, even night rests are frequently challenged. Achieving extra moments of spiritual tranquillity is a blessing for all. Buddhists, monks and priests have means and experience acquiring the spiritual tranquillity. *Qi Gong*, *Tai Chi* and Yoga practices aim at the same achievement. Through the practice of stretching and controlled breathing, that state of mind is expected to automatically come. Is this a myth? Should one need to reach the mental state of a fervent religious follower before one reaches such a spiritual state? May be the extraordinary neurological inputs from stretching and controlled respiration are the hidden benefactors pushing toward the state of tranquillity. Firstly, stretching controls any pain (through the Gate theory), eliminates stiffness, relaxes the musculoskeletal components, thus removes adverse somatic inputs and initiates pleasant humoral exchanges within the brain. Secondly, the controlled breathing mobilises independent autonomic nervous pathways which help to adjust contradicting physiological activities at humoral levels. The outcome of the unusual input from the two normally uncoordinated systems of neurological activities could be a novel state of harmony between the body and mind.

With this obviously optimistic, yet over-simplified concept in mind, one could confidently start one's own personal practice of Natural Healing using any form of *Qi Gong*, *Tai Chi* or Yoga. One may even invent his own practice as long as the activities consist of stretching, controlled breathing and meditation.

How is *Qi Gong, Tai Chi* and Yoga different from aerobic exercises? Aerobic exercises aim at the training of skeletal muscles which directly pull on the joints in the normal day to day fashion. As much energy is needed, oxygen consumption needs to be sharply increased. The result is a need for a parallel increase in the efficacy of the lungs and the heart. The rationale of aerobic exercises, therefore, is to engage in a comprehensive training of musculo — skeleto — cardio — pulmonary function (Irwin and Olmstead, 2007). All these are normal day-to-day physiological functions. In contrast, *Qi Gong, Tai Chi* and Yoga consist of static exercises coupled with a variable amount of dynamic moves. A lot of unusual, extraordinary neurological stimulations are elicited through the stretching and stimulation of muscles and ligaments. The controlled respirations elicit autonomic nervous stimulations which again do not happen normally. Henceforth, the mental state of tranquillity obtained through *Qi Gong, Tai Chi* and Yoga is something unimaginable for anyone doing strenuous aerobic exercises.

Aerobic exercises have limitations, not only during performance, but also in the long term. Over strenuous musculoskeletal training is going to damage the joints. In fact, biomechanical studies have indicated that if jogging exceeds the frequency of one mile per day and three times per week, cartilage damages will be inevitable. In the case of *Qi Gong, Tai Chi* and Yoga, limitations on the physiological ability during the training are virtually unknown, and in the long term, the joints involved do not suffer any threatening damages.

What about other means advocated for the practice of Natural Healing like special food and botanicals?

It is true that Natural Healing involves food and botanicals in both European and Oriental Practices. Food and botanicals are considered "natural" because they occur in Nature in spite of the fact that feeding individuals with special purposes do not appear that "natural". When the oldest Chinese medicine classic *Ne-jing* discussed Natural Healing, only stretching, controlled breathing and meditation were emphasised again and again. Use of other means like botanicals are additional measures created by subsequent clinicians when either exercises fails to give the desirable effects or more rapid responses are needed for various reasons.

Qi Gong, and *Tai Chi* could therefore be taken as the essential practices leading to Natural Healing and Longevity while botanicals can be used as supportive, secondary tools.

Exercises have long been known to be good and effective means of self-administered treatment, not only for physical strengthening but also in attempts to sooth the mind. Indeed, many past and current studies have given good evidences to the objective reasoning and physiological changes behind the simple practice. Practising meditations under various artificial initiations, have attracted a lot of attention as an effective means of promoting mental health.

When Yoga and *Qi Gong* both require sustained stretching and controlled breathing, leading gradually into a state of meditation, the self-initiating activities could be triggering off combined or synergistic effects derived from different levels of neurological activities. Harvard University has conducted a survey on Yoga practitioners in 2008, and found that they were mainly people (woman more than men) who were suffering from musculoskeletal or mental disturbances. The survey indicated that 5.1% of US populations have used Yoga for health in the past 12 months, representing 10.4 million individuals. The data gives sufficient support for further recommendation on the popular use of the simple safe practice, so easily learned and adopted by all (Saper *et al.*, 2004). When Mayo Clinic staff made wide propaganda on exercises, using this slogan: "Depression and Anxiety: Exercises ease Symptoms" and giving clear explanations and instruction on Yoga, they were well accepted (Mayo Clinic, 2014).

Given the great similarities between Yoga and *Qi Gong*, there might be a great justification for exploring the two systems of therapies together, when they are recommended as alternative treatments for a holistic body–mind resolution against stress, anxiety and depression. Yoga or *Qi Gong* is a safe prescription for healthy living and provides a rich ground for harmonised human existence basing on the mind's self-regulatory processes against mental stresses. The two alternative therapies may control mental health disruptions like anxiety and depression, helping to maintain an ideal quality of life (Rime *et al.*, 2012).

The author is neither an expert on Yoga nor *Qi Gong*. He is a practising surgeon researching on Alternative Medicine as a supplementary support to mainline scientific allopathic medicine. He does practice *Qi Gong* and has studied Yoga superficially. He realises Yoga and *Qi Gong* could both be excellent additional support for physical and mental health. While searching for literal evidences to illustrate the value of Yoga and *Qi Gong* for mental health, he found many convincing conceptual literature, superficial in the scientific sense, but well-covers the breadth that is required for those interested to know more about Yoga and *Qi Gong*. Readers need not be disappointed with the lack of specific evidences on specific mental diseases, because Yoga and *Qi Gong* are meant to be supplementary, not replacing the conventional specialist treatment. Likewise, strict scientific data like hormones and transmitters might have been included in some of the reports, however, for the general proof of concept, being too specific might lead to a different direction.

References

Arias, A.J., Steinberg, K., Banga, A. and Trestman, R.L. (2006). Systematic review of the efficacy of meditation techniques as treatments for medical illness. *J. Altern. Complement. Med.* **12**(8), 817–832.

Astin, J.A., Shapiro, S.L., Eisenberg, D.M. and Forys, K.L. (2003). Mind-body medicine: state of the science, implications for practice. *J. Am. Board. Fam. Pract.* **16**(2), 131–147.

Astsumi, K. (2007). Integrative approach towards "healthy aging". In: *Proceedings of "Inter Natural Symposium on Healthy Aging"*. Tokyo University Press, Tokyo, pp. 2–5.

Brevetti, G. and Schiano, V. (2006). Cellular adhesion molecules and peripheral arterial disease. *Vasc. Med.* **11**(1), 39–47.

Brown, R.P. and Gerbarg, P.L. (2005a). Sudarshan Kriya yogic breathing in the treatment of stress, anxiety, and depression: part 1–neurophysiologic model. *J. Altern. Complement. Med.* **11**(1), 189–201.

Brown, R.P. and Gerbarg, P.L. (2005b). Sudarshan Kriya yogic breathing in the treatment of stress, anxiety, and depression: part II — clinical application and guidelines. *J. Altern. Complement. Med.* **11**(4), 711–717.

Chang, C. and Wai, S. (1997). *Tai Chi* and physiology of middle and old aged people. *J. Binzhou Med. Coll.* **20**(5), 505.

Chang, W.C., Zhung, T.B. and Wu, C.H. (2006). *Qi gong* and cognitive changes. *Chin. J.Behav. Med. Sci.* **15**(9), 827–828.

Chen, J.H. (1998). Natural healing and *Tai Chi*. *World Sci. Tech.* **5**, 15–18.

Chen, M.K. (2009). *Qi gong* and osteoporosis. *Consuma. Guide Tech. Forum* **10**, 217–218.

Chen, W.Z. and Chang, T. (2002). *Qi gong* and hand temperature. *J. Int. Soc. Life Inform. Sci.* **20**(2), 707–110.

Du, S.W., Chang, C.L. and Wang, S. (2006). *Qi gong* and cardiac function of middle and old age people. *Chin J. Sports Med.* **25**(6), 721–726.

Green, D.J. and Blankshy, B.A. (1996). Control skeletal muscle blood flow during dynamic exercise. *J. Sports Med.* **21**, 119–146.

Griffith, J.M., Hasley, J.P., Liu, H., Severn, D.G., Conner, L.H. and Adler, L.E. (2008). *Qi gong* Stress reduction in hospital staff. *J. Altern. a compl. Med.* **14**(8), 939–945.

Harvard Mental Health Letter, April 2009. *Yoga for anxiety and depression.* Accessed Jan 20, 2014. https://www.health.harvard.edu/newsletters/Harvard_Mental_Health_Letter/2009/April/Yoga-for-anxiety-and-depression

Hsu, H.F. (1986). *Qi Gong* and immunological indices. *Qi Gong* **6**, 279–283.

Hsu, S.W. and Wang, W.J. (1986). *Tai Chi* and internal secretion. *China J. Phys. Med.* **5**(3), 150–153.

Huang, J. (2009). History, current situation and future of stretching exercises in disease prevention. *J. Beijing Univ. Tradit. Chin. Med.* **32**(9), 586–589.

Huang, Y.H., Leong, Y.F. and Jim, C.L. (2001). *Tai Chi* influence on elderly people's serum anti oxidants. *Occup. Health Inj.* **16**(3), 139–141.

Irwin, M.R. and Olmstead, R. (2007). Augmenting immune responses to varicella zoster virus in older adults: A randomized controlled trial of *Tai Chi*. *J. Am. Geriatr. Soc.* **55**, 511–517.

Janakiramaiah, N., Gangadhar, B.N., Naga Venkatesha Murthy, P.J., Harish, M.G., Subbakrishna, D.K. and Vedamurthachar, A. (2000). Antidepressant efficacy of Sudarshan Kriya Yoga (SKY) in melancholia: a randomized comparison with electroconvulsive therapy (ECT) and imipramine. *J. affect. Disord.* **57**(1), 255–259.

Ji, L.Z. (1994a). Natural healing in Chinese medicine. *Beijing Chin. Med. J.* **1**, 62–63.

Ji, L.Z. (1994b). Natural healing in Chinese medicine. *Beijing Chin. Med. J.* **2**, 62–63.

Ji, L.Z. (1994c). Natural healing in Chinese medicine. *Beijing Chin. Med. J.* **3**, 61–63.

Ji, L.Z. (1994d). Natural healing in Chinese medicine. *Beijing Chin. Med. J.* **4**, 63–65.

Ji, L.Z. (1994e). Natural healing in Chinese medicine. *Beijing Chin. Med. J.* **5**, 63–64.

Jones, B.M. (2001). Change in cytokine production in healthy subjects practicing *Qi gong*: A pilot study. *J. Complement. Altern. Med.* **1**, 8–10.

Jorm, A.F., Christensen, H., Griffiths, K.M., Parslow, R.A., Rodgers, B. and Blewitt, K.A. (2004). Effectiveness of complementary and self-help treatments for anxiety disorders. *Med. J. Aust.* **181**(7 Suppl), S29–S46.

Jouper, J. and Johansson, M. (2013). *Qi gong* and mindfulness-based mood recovery: exercise experiences from a single case. *J. Bodyw. M. Ther.* **17**(1), 69–76.

Khalsa, S.B. (2004). Yoga as a Therapeutic Intervention: a bibliometric analysis of published research studies. *Indian J. of Physiol. Pharmacol.* **48**(3), 269–285.

Kirkwood, G., Rampes, H., Tuffrey, V., Richardson, J., Pikington, K. and Ramaratnam, S. (2005). Yoga for anxiety: a systematic review of the research evidence. *Br. J. Sports Med.* **39**(12), 884–891.

Krisanaprakornkit, T., Krisanaprakornkit, W., Piyavhatkul, N. and Laopaiboon, M. (2006). Meditation therapy for anxiety disorders. *Cochrane Database Syst. Rev.* CD004998.

Lafferty, W.E., Downey, L., McCarty, R.L., Standish, L.J., Standish, L.J. and Patrick, D.L. (2006). Evaluating CAM treatment at the end of life: a review of clinical trials for massage and meditation. *Complement. Ther. Med.* **14**(2), 100–112.

Lewicki, E. (1988). Effects of maximal physical exercise on T lymphocyte subpopulations and on interleukin 1 (IL 1) and interleukin 2 (IL 2) production *in vitro*. *Int. J. Sports Med.* **9**(2), 114–117.

Li, S.C. and Chu, W.C. (2008). Recent scientific research on *Qi gong* in Japan. *Rep. Relat. Chin. Med. Outside China* **25**(5), 276–279.

Liang, X.S. (2005). Natural healing. *J. Xiaolin Tai Chi* **1**, 53.

Lic, S. (2003). Four ways of natural healing I and II. *Natural Healing Monthly* (養生月刊) Feb. & Mar.

Lin, W.N. and Wang, W.T. (2009). Natural healing and type 2 diabetes. *Beijing J. Tradit. Chin. Med.* **28**(1), 9–12.

Liu, H.F., An, H.Y. and Mung, F.Y. (2008). Research on impact of health *Qi gong* (Baduanjin) on mental health of medical college students. *Med. Soc.* **21**(8), 63–64.

Lui, S.S., Yi, H.A. and Chen, C.Y. (2001). *Tai Chi* and cardio pulmonary function. *Modern Rehabil.* **5**(6), 64–65.

Maki, B.E. (1990). Aging and postural control. *J. Am. Geriatr. Soc.* **38**(1), 1–9.

Mao, C. (2002). Influence of exercise training on elderly people with borderline hypertension. *Chin. J. Clin. Rehabil.* **6**(11), 1673–1676.

Mayo Clinic (2014). Depression and anxiety: exercise eases symptoms. Accessed Jan 20, 2014. http://www.mayoclinic.com.

Motoyama, M. and Sunami, Y. (1998). Low intensity aerobic training in elderly hypertensive people. *J. Med. Sci. Sport Exerc.* **30**(6), 818–813.

Penman, S., Cohen, M., Stevens, P. and Jackson, S. (2012). Yoga in Australia: results of a national survey. *Int. J. Yoga* **5**(2), 92–101.

Pilkington, K., Kirkwood, G., Rampes, H. and Richardson, J. (2005). Yoga for depression: the research evidence. *J. Affect Disord.* **89**(1–3), 13–24.

Rime, J., Dwan, K., Lawlor, D.A., Greig, C.A., McMurdo, M., Morley, W. and Mead, G.E. (2012). Exercise for depression. *Cochrane Database Syst. Rev.* CD004366.

Saper, R.B., Eisenberg, D.M., Davis, R.B., Culpepper, L. and Phillip, R.S. (2004). Prevalence and patterns of adult Yoga use in United States: results of a natural survey. *Altern. Ther. Health. Med.* **10**(2), 44–49.

Shao, L. and Zhou, Y. (2008). *Tai Chi* and work injury back pain. *J. Shanxi Normal Univ.* **36**(5), 35–36.

Shi, J. (2005). *Qigong* and mental health. *J. Xianning College* **25**(6), 110–113.

Shi, A.Q., Li, A.M., Wang, G.L., Xiang, H.P. and Lei, B. (2005). Influence of older's psychology and physiology by practicing *Yijinjing* (Fitness *Qigong*). *Journal of Chengdu Sport University* **31**(3), 95–97.

Si, H.Y. (2006). Fitness *Qi gong* of health. *Chin. J. Clin. Rehabil.* **10**(47), 145–147.

Suen, L.F., Lui, S.P. and Hsu, J.H. (1989). Clinical evaluation of declining cognitive power — application in research of TCM. *J. Integr. Med.* **9**, 203–207.

Taggart, H.M., Arslanian, C.L., Bae, S. and Singh, K. (2003). Effects of *Tai Chi* exercise on fibromyalgia symptoms and health-related quality of life. *Orthop. Nurs.* **22**(5), 353–360.

Tao, G.S. and Tung, W. (1988). Indices of aging. *China J. Geriatr. Med.* **7**(3), 167–172.

Tsang, Y.K. and Chow, S.C. (2005). Natural healing and physiological changes of middle and elderly age people. *J. Beijing Sport Univ.* **28**(9), 1206–1209.

Wang, Y. (2002). *Tai Chi* and hypertension of the elderly. *J. Marshal Art Sci.* **1**(4), 47–52.

Wang, C.J. (2003). *Tai Chi* and interleukins. *J. Shantung Inst. Sport* **19**(2), 48–30.

Wang, L. and Xiang, L.J. (2006). Principles of Chinese medicine and *Tai Chi. J. Shanxi Coll. Tradit. Chin. Med.* **29**(5), 4–6.

Wang, C. (2007). Natural healing in Chinese medicine. *Scholast. Rev.* (學習時報) **7**, 23–25.

Wang, T., Lu, W. and Wu, Z.Y. (2007). Hypertension rehabilitated with walking or *Tai Chi. Modern Prevent. Med.* **34**(18), 3535–3543.

Wang, K.H. (2008). Historical changes of natural healing exercises in China. *Sports Culture J.* **3** (體育文化專刊).

Whelton, S.P. (2002). Effects of aerobic exercise on blood pressure: A meta-analysis of randomized controlled trials. *Ann. Int. Med.* **136**, 493–503.

Won, J.C. (2004). Natural healing and *Tai Chi. Anhui J. Sport Tech.* **9**, 93–95.

Won, X.S. (2008). Natural healing review. *Tai Chi Rev.* **11**, 29–30.

Yang, W. (2001). Natural healing and *Tai Chi. J. Fujian Coll. Tradit. Chin. Med.* **2**, 56–57.

Yen, Y. (2009). *Qi gong* influence on serum fatty acids. *J. Liaoning Normal Univ.* **32**(3), 356–358.

Yi, L.O. (2008). *Tai Chi* and elderly health. *China J. Health Psychol.* **16**(4), 477–478.

Yi, X.K. (2007). Natural healing in Chinese medicine. *World Health Digest* **4**, 269–270.

Zhai, X.Y. (2006). Investigation on cultivating mental hygiene with gymnastic *Qi gong* practice. *Journal of Henan University of Chinese Medicine* **21**(3), 47–48.

Chapter 8

Ayurveda in India

Debashis Panda and Ping-Chung Leung

Abstract

Ayurveda is considered to be the oldest system of medical care in human history. Now Ayurveda is gaining popularity in towns and cities. The Ministry of Ayurveda, Yoga, Unani, Siddha and Homeopathy (AYUSH) has been established under the independent charge of the Minister of State. It supports the establishment of infrastructures like hospitals, clinics, and community centres. Many influential Indians think that integrating the ancient medical system of Ayurveda with modern allopathic medicine is the key to providing universal health care.

Keywords: Ayurveda; Ayurvedic Medicine; Ayurveda, Yoga, Unani, Siddha and Homeopathy (AYUSH); Allopathic Medicine.

8.1 Introduction

Ayurveda in India is considered to be the oldest system of medical care in human history, taken to be 5,000 years old with good documents of around 3,000 years. Today, it is not difficult to review its history, principles and current status, which should include government administrative management, education, service and research activities (University of Maryland Medical Center, 2015).

Many influential Indians, including Prime Minister Narendra Modi, think that integrating the ancient medical system of Ayurveda with modern allopathic medicine is the key to providing universal health care. The fact is, practitioners of traditional medicine (TM) remain the primary health care providers for millions of people in the rural areas of India. Ayurvedic practitioners prescribe individual preventive and curative interventions, such as herbal combinations, dietary control, exercises, manual therapies, Yoga and life-style recommendations. Like everywhere in the world, allopathic medicine has made great contributions in life-threatening areas like injuries, infections and pathologies with straightforward targets. However, difficulties and controversies remain plentiful in the growing epidemics of non-communicable and life-style related diseases, which deserve to be explored. The World Health Organization launched its Traditional Medicine Strategy 2014–2023 which aims to support member states to develop policies on the strengthening of the role of TM in keeping populations healthy (WHO, 2013; CCIM, 2012a, 2012b).

Since coming to power in 2014, Modi has done much to focus on making traditional forms of medicine mainstream. The Ministry of Ayurveda, Yoga, Unani, Siddha and Homeopathy (AYUSH) has been established under the independent charge of the Minister of State. The National AYUSH Mission was launched in September 2014 to complement allopathic medicine, especially in remote rural areas with poor access to modern health facilities. It supports the establishment of infrastructures like hospitals, clinics, and community centres.

Ayurveda is also gaining popularity in towns and cities. Advocates consider Ayurvedic medicine less technology and infrastructure intensive and therefore relies on knowledge and human capital for its implementation (Furst *et al.*, 2011; Chopra *et al.*, 2013).

A review on the changing scenario for promotion and development of Ayurveda has shown many reliable data. The 2012 data showed that in India, there are 2,420 Ayurveda hospitals with about 42,000 beds and 15,000 dispensaries. There are 320 Ayurveda educational institutes and 7,700 Ayurveda drug factories. The number of registered Ayurvedic practitioners is just short of half a million (Narahari *et al.*, 2013).

Traditional Ayurvedic service is growing its popularity under special areas like chronic pain, management and rehabilitation. Some established modern hospitals are setting up Ayurvedic consultation centres, while others are starting clinical trials. For example, two randomised controlled trials are under way to test whether Ayurveda has clinical benefits for the management of mucositis during radiation therapy for head and neck cancer and for the management of side effects and quality of life in patients with breast cancer undergoing chemo-radiotherapy. Each trial has 60 patients and will be completed by the end of 2016.

Ayurvedic practices are believed to benefit patients. A 2011 double blind, randomised, placebo controlled pilot study of 43 patients found that an Ayurvedic herbal compound was just as effective treating rheumatoid arthritis symptoms as methotrexate but with fewer adverse events.

A non-randomised interventional study on community level morbidity control of lymphedema in two districts of southern India where lymphatic filariasis is endemic showed that self-care and treatments that integrated Ayurveda were possible in village settings. A total of 730 of 1,008 patients completed three and half months' follow-up and showed a statistically significant reduction in the volume of their lower limbs. The AYUSH Research Councils, which have 81 research centres across the country, are collaborating with other institutes on clinical trials on the safety and efficacy of drugs so as to meet the US and European Union regulations.

Darshan Shankar, vice chancellor of the Transdisciplinary University (Institute of Transdisciplinary Health Sciences and Technology) in Bangalore, suggested setting up a fourth tier of self-help health management that would not be institutionally driven like primary, secondary and tertiary health care, but where the providers are millions of households. The traditional Indian medicine system has many simple and cost effective solutions for common ailments, prevention and wellness (Bhandari, 2015; CCIM, 2012b).

Health activists argue that a more patient-centred approach to healthcare is needed if universal healthcare in India is to become a reality. Allopathic treatments have provided longevity, and Ayurveda can add quality to this prolonged life. The government needs to implement a policy framework whereby integration of TM systems with allopathy is validated (Bhandari, 2015; CCIM, 2012b).

8.2 What the Indian Government has Done for Ayurveda

One Chinese scholar has done extensive exploration on the Indian Government's policy on the promotion of Ayurveda. The summary of her work gives a concise account of the situation in 2012.

Service Statistics

AYUSH hospitals in India amount to 27.5% of all hospitals, providing 58,000 beds which represent 9.7% of all hospital beds.

AYUSH clinicians amount to 720,000 which is 43.7%.

In the rural areas, community set-ups providing AYUSH services are plentiful, well superseding those providing modern services (51.6% versus 35.7%)

It is estimated that there are 25.9 AYUSH hospitals every 10 million people; 0.3 AYUSH clinics per 10,000 people; 0.5 hospital beds per 10,000 people and 5.9 AYUSH clinicians per 10,000 people.

In 2012, there has been a flourish of new AYUSH hospitals and clinics, amounting to 90% of overall new hospitals and 89.8% of overall new clinics in India.

Provision of Human Resources

In order to rapidly satisfy the expanding Ayurveda service, India restored the old system apprenticeship, so that a twin system of manpower provision, institutionally qualified and non-institutionally qualified AYUSH clinicians coexist. It is believed that this twin system not only takes care of the manpower shortage, but also help to better maintain the traditional AYUSH philosophy.

Education

Since 2003, there has been an annual increase in the number of student admissions for undergraduate study in Ayurveda medicine and number of institutes providing Ayurveda courses. In 2002, a total of 260 Ayurveda institutes are taking 10,000 new students annually. There are also technical schools producing lower level Ayurveda medical graduates. Obviously, government efforts put on education for modern medicine are well matched by the traditional stream.

Research

The emphasis has been put on clinical effects for the improvement of health services.

Industrial activities

The industrial productions are mainly raw herbs or proprietary herbal drugs, the profit margins of which are limited. With the increasing demand on quality production, standard GMP (good manufacture practice) set-ups are increasing at the expense of small industries being eliminated.

8.3 Continuous Support Given to Ayurvedic Medicine

In the early' 20s, the city of Bombay had only one medical college, the Grant Medical College, and JJ Hospital to cater to the health care of Bombay. India was under British rule and naturally the college was managed by the British. No Indian doctors were appointed irrespective of their academic background and experience. Local nationalistic leaders felt that the city should have a medical college that is established only with the help of locally generated funds without taking any help from the British rulers. Through donations from the Tilak Swaraj Funds, on the fourth of September 1921, the National Medical College was established. This College started functioning at the Victoria Cross Lane, Byculla. The founding fathers wanted to train doctors who could serve not only through hospitals, but would also reach out to the community. Ayurveda became an obligatory part of the curriculum.

The Ayurvidyavardhini Trust was then established. It is a public charitable trust later registered under Bombay Public Charitable Trust Act 1950, with an objective to elevate the status of Ayurveda as a primary health care system. The trust undertakes activities for promotion and implementation of fundamental and applied research to Ayurveda. It also aims to hold lectures, exhibition, public meetings, classes and conferences to teach and train students of Ayurveda and modern medicine in interdisciplinary approach.

8.4 Dr. Sharadini Dahanukar Advanced Centre for Ayurveda Research, Training & Services

In 2001, the Advanced Centre for Ayurveda Research, Training & Services was established at the Department of Clinical Pharmacology, TN Medical College, Mumbai. It is one of the rare Centres in India situated in a Modern health care hospital, rendering Ayurvedic services and performing advanced research. The activities of this Centre are primarily supported by the Ayurvidyavardhini, a charitable trust.

The objectives of the Centre are:

- To generate a strong evidence base for Ayurvedic principles, concepts and therapies.
- To explore and develop new drugs taking leads from Ayurveda.
- To build and strengthen human resources in the field of Ayurvedic research by conducting various training courses.
- To strengthen pharmacovigilance in Ayurveda.
- To educate lay people about the concepts and therapies of Ayurveda.

Research Activities include:

- *Prakriti* and their correlation with biomarkers and candidate genes.
- Establishing standards for various bhasmas and exploring their efficacy and safety.
- Undertaking clinical trials to evaluate the efficacy and mechanism of action of Ayurvedic therapeutic procedures (*Panchakarma*).
- Developing new drug molecules taking leads from Ayurvedic pharmacopoeia particularly for diabetes and tuberculosis.
- Establishing simple bioassays to evaluate activity of plants, which can be further used for bioassay guided standardisation and fractionation of the plants.

- Setting-up of in-house quality control (QC) systems for plants.
- Pharmacovigilance of Ayurvedic remedies.

The Centre offers training in varied fields:

- Teaching M.Sc. and Ph.D. courses in Applied Biology which are recognised by the University of Mumbai.
- Externship provision for foreign students.
- Conducting training courses on a regular basis in Clinical Pharmacology of TM for modern medicine fraternity and Clinical Research Methodology for Ayurvedic scholars.
- Organising Update Ayurveda, an International Conference, every four years that aims at providing a single platform for Ayurvedic research work being carried out at national and international level.

The Centre (situated in a tertiary care hospital) provides quality services such as:

- An Ayurvedic outpatient department that caters to around 1,500 patients a year free of cost.
- *Panchakarma* (Ayurvedic therapeutic procedures) unit on an out patient basis at a minimal cost. This centre has been established with support from the Department of AYUSH, Govt. of India.
- Specialised Cell to monitor and document adverse drug reactions reported with the use of Traditional or Alternative therapies and detect contamination/adulteration of Ayurvedic drugs with steroids and heavy metals.
- Protocol drafting for different phases of drug development, data management and analysis for Ayurvedic Pharmaceutical companies.
- Undertaking Corporate-sponsored research projects.

8.5 Concern with Safety

The FDA in US cautioned against the use of Ayurvedic products in 2008 because a study through the routine screening of such products demonstrated that one-fifth of US-manufactured and Indian manufactured

Ayurvedic products bought on the Internet contained detectable lead, mercury or arsenic to well above acceptable levels.

It is true that Ayurvedic medicine favours the addition of metallic components particularly items belonging to the *Bhasmas* category. However, experts argue that *Bhasmas* are generally safe drugs for human consumption in spite of the presence of seemingly toxic elements and compounds. Nevertheless, more systematic Nanomaterialistic investigations are recommended for gaining the complete and reliable picture on the composition-processing-structural changes-and effectiveness of the Bhasmas (Adhikari, 2014).

References

Adhikari, R. (2014). Ayurvedic Bhasmas: overview on nanomaterialistic aspects, applications, and perspectives. *Adv. Exp. Med. Biol.* **807,** 23–32.

Bhandari, N. (2015). Is ayurveda the key to universal healthcare in India? *BMJ.* **350,** 1–3.

Central Council of Indian Medicine (CCIM) (2012a). *Indian Medicine Central Council (Minimum Standards of Education in Indian Medicine) (amendment).* https://ccimindia.org/cc_act_ug_regulations_2012.php

Central Council of Indian Medicine (CCIM) (2012b). *Notification, 16 March.* http://ccimindia.org/ayurveda-pg-reg.php

Chopra, A., Saluja, M., Tillu, G. *et al.* (2013). Ayurvedic medicine offers a good alternative to glucosamine and celecoxib in the treatment of symptomatic knee osteoarthritis: a randomized, double-blind, controlled equivalence drug trial. *Rheumatology,* **52,** 1408–1417.

Furst, D.E. Venkatraman, M.M., McGann, M. *et al.* (2011). Double-blind, randomized, controlled, pilot study comparing classic ayurvedic medicine, methotrexate, and their combination in rheumatoid arthritis. *J. Clin. Rheumatol.* **17,** 185–192.

Narahari, S.R. Bose, K.S., Aggithaya, M.G. *et al.* (2013). Community level morbidity control of lymphedema using self care and integrative treatment in two lymphatic filariasis endemic districts of South India: a non randomized interventional study. *Trans. R. Soc. Trop. Med. Hyg.* **107,** 566–577.

University of Maryland Medical Center (2015). *Ayurveda.* Available at http://umm.edu/health/medical/altmed/treatment/ayurveda.

World Health Organization (WHO) (2013). *WHO traditional medicine strategy: 2014–2023.* www.who.int/medicines/publications/traditional/trm_strategy14_23/en/.

Chapter 9

Traditional Medicine in China

Ping-Chung Leung

Abstract

Traditional Chinese Medicine (TCM) has always been the main offer of health promotion and medical care in China. The long and fruitful history has greatly helped to maintain the high degree of acceptance to traditional medicine (TM) which perpetuates until today. This chapter concisely introduces the current status of TM in China.

Keywords: Traditional Chinese Medicine (TCM); Apprenticeship Training; Allopathic Medicine; Chinese Medicine Services; Dietary Supplements; Integration.

9.1 Introduction

With the over 3,000 years of history, Traditional Chinese Medicine (TCM) has always been the main offer of health promotion and medical care throughout China until less than 90 years ago, when allopathic medicine was gradually introduced from Europe. The long and fruitful history has greatly helped to maintain the high degree of acceptance to traditional medicine (TM) which perpetuates until today (Stone, 2008).

The successes and contributions of allopathic medicine, however, must have down-graded the trust and, with the increasing investments on modern medicine, together with the fascinating technological supports enjoyed by modern medicine, one witnesses a decline in the trust and stagnation of development in the traditional field. Thus, TM has receded from the mainline to the supplementary area of service and professional recognition (Bivins, 2008).

9.2 Education in Traditional Chinese Medicine

After the communists' takeover, the traditional way of teaching in Chinese medicine has advanced from the old apprenticeship to proper professional institutional education. Currently, there are 32 Chinese Medicine Universities and 52 Comprehensive Universities offering herbal pharmacology or Chinese medicine courses. The total number of Chinese medicine students is estimated to be around 270,000 while senior respectable Chinese medicine experts are still taking graduates under apprenticeship training.

In spite of the formalisation of undergraduate training and the mounting increases in educational resources for TCMs, it has been observed that the general quantity of the graduates is apparently downgrading. The problems include: a declining interest on the classical concepts and philosophy, obsolete teaching methodology and marginalisation of traditional classic volumes. Students are receiving low-quality clinical training while their knowledge about medicinal plants and dried herbs are limited. Another obvious threat to young students' pursuing the Chinese medicine practitioner's career exists in the rather narrow pathway of clinical commitment. It is not uncommon to find graduates entering completely different fields. One way to overcome the declining popularity is taking the form of integrated service, combining allopathic and TM in joint services. In view of the lack of clear division of labour, integration would remain unclear, while the overwhelming authoritative scientific approaches of allopathic medicine would not allow proper sharing of efforts (Xu, 2001; MOH Singapore, 1995).

9.3 Traditional Chinese Medicine Services

TCM services are widespread. The National Policy, for over half a century, has been insisting on at least 20% of national resources to be given to

TCM. Regarding infrastructure, over 3,000 municipal level hospitals for Chinese medicine are established. Over 330,000 beds are provided, over 160 specialties are allocated. 90% of comprehensive hospitals are in possession of special Chinese medicine services. The number of registered Chinese medicine practitioner ranged from 520,000 (certificate) to 237,000 (fully registered). Over 240 million out-patient visit per year have been recorded. 18.5% emergency care are provided by traditional practitioners.

The low cost required for Chinese medicine consultation has helped to maintain its popularity. On the other hand, the limited resources would have restricted research and development. The Health Policymakers have well protected the rapid, deterioration of trust. However, without making clear recommendations on the selective utilisation of TM today, allopathic medicine has much stronger attractions. The general protective measures fail to convince the patient–public on the most sensible utilisation of the traditional service (MOH China, 1995; Wong *et al.*, 1993).

9.4 Research on Traditional Chinese Medicine

The strong traditional use of proprietary herbal medicine has helped to maintain a rather prosperous market. Herbal items on sale are usually those handed down since hundreds or thousands of years. Attempts to give modern evidence to their current uses are scanty. Though unusual, innovative new creations are available, not many of them would go through evidence-based investigations. Clinical trials on new applications are reported, but it is well-known that most, if not all, of these trials are of poor qualities.

Pharmacologists interested in Chinese medicine are following the only research direction of drug discovery. Infrastructures designed for research on TM are plentiful (over 180) and an estimated 30,000 researchers are involved.

Isolate groups are trying to work out scientific supports for the traditional concepts of TM which are often more philosophical than scientific or technical. As of date, little successful results are available.

The Industrial side of TM appears to be brighter since the export of herbal medicine and related products has been increasing in the past 20 years at a rate of about 20% per year. Amidst this optimism, the deteriorating quality of herbs has already emerged as a real threat. The causative factors like environmental pollution, over-cultivation, adulterations and poor quality controls, are all contributive (Leung and Wong, 2002; Jonas, 1998).

9.5 Safety of Chinese Medicine

Is the use of Chinese medicinal material safe?

Experienced TCM practitioners assure us that the hundreds of years of utilisation have given us a vivid picture of safety. The unsafe items are all known and properly recorded so that they need to be used with utmost care and be prescribed by herbal experts. Currently, Chinese medicinal herbs in common use have been categorised into three groups, *viz.* those strictly for drug use, those for both drug and supplement and those for supplement and food (NCCIH, 2009). The three categories clearly give indications for related safety.

However, we do note that from time to time, reports give striking information about poison cases after consumption of certain items in the drug or drug-supplement category of medicinal Chinese herbs. The explanation given is usually illegal adulteration or unprofessional preparation or processing of the raw herbs. In spite of the obviously over-simplistic explanations, the worry about safety related to Chinese herbs is in no way changed.

In fact, herbal experts used to comment: "all medicinal material could be considered harmful if consumed for prolonged periods" This concept does help, particularly for those chronic users.

When medicinal herbs are marketed as food or food supplement, consumers might form their subjective view of safety, thus might cause varieties of unsafe situations.

The fact is some Chinese herbal products may be safe, but others may not be. There have been reports of products being contaminated with drugs, toxins, or heavy metals or not containing the listed ingredients. Some of the herbs used in Chinese medicine can interact with drugs, can have serious side effects, or may be unsafe for people with certain medical conditions. For example the Chinese herb ephedra (*ma huang*) has been linked to serious health complications, including heart attack and stroke. In 2004, the FDA banned the sale of ephedra-containing dietary supplements, but the ban does not apply to TCM remedies.

Herbal medicines used in TCM are sometimes marketed in the United States as dietary supplements. The US Food and Drug Administration (FDA) regulations for dietary supplements are not the same as those for prescription of over-the-counter drugs; in general, the regulations for dietary supplements are less stringent. For example, manufacturers do not have to prove to the FDA that most claims made for dietary supplements are valid; if the product were a drug, they would have to provide proof (NCCIH, 2009).

A logical way to ensure safety from the position of the user could be to use with extreme caution the herbs that are recommended for drug only, preferably after approval by herbal clinicians. For the researcher on the provision of health supplement or proprietary drugs, it might be wise of them to totally avoid that category.

9.6 Globalisation of Chinese Medicine

The scientific and technological advancements of allopathic medicine would have left little room for the development of TCM, had it not been complicated pathologies blocking the over-all satisfactions. Selective dissatisfied patients start to look for “alternative” or “complementary” solutions. Acupuncture is highly regarded and popular as a means to control pain and neurologically related symptoms. Other areas of Chinese medicine are gradually gaining attention, and medical groups are organised to explore the various means and justifications for application (Cheng and Sze, 2015).

Within China itself, advocates on the integration of modern and TM have retained their momentum although critiques tend to be sceptical in that integration often which means giving up the traditional concepts and just using the herbal medicine as supplements to the allopathic treatment. This attitude has been taken to the extreme so that scientists openly advocated in 2007 that TM should be eliminated.

In fact, towards the end of the Qing Dynasty, and during the Nationalist China a few episodes of similar nature have occurred when science and technology was introduced to China from Europe and when antagonists exaggerated certain hazardous social events like herbal toxicities. All aggressive attempts to removal TCM were short-lived as could be expected. The Centuries of cultural respect and contributions would remain as strong as ever. Indeed, after every negative move (which is apparently out of the context) supportive, promotions would be organised. In the years following 2007, the Ministry of China has done a lot to further endorse the proper value of TCM (Leung, 2008). In 2008, which was labelled as the Year of Chinese medicine, big cities in China took turns to host seminars and conference on different health topics related to the philosophy and practice of Chinese medicine. More importantly, the People's Congress, which is the Highest Authority on Legislation, is prepared to pass a Legal Document on Chinese medicine.

9.7 Chinese Medicine Under the Protection of Peoples Congress

In December 2015, the Minister responsible for the planning and development of Chinese medicine was entrusted the role of giving the final explanations in the next standing committee meeting about the Legislation on Chinese medicine as a uniquely important event in the People's Congress. This would mark the final preparation for the legalisation of Chinese medicine which has been put under the National Agenda for at least 30 years.

The Draft Legislation consists of 46 items, divided into eight chapters, *viz.* General Statements, Chinese Medicine Services, Chinese Medicine Development, Education and Training, Cultural Heritage and Innovation, Protection and Promotion, Legal Responsibilities and Attachments. It has been pointed out that in spite of the popular use of Chinese medicine and historical importance, four major problems exist. They are: (i) Declining service ability and failure to establish the unique nature of Chinese medicine; (ii) The existing system of regulation on the quality of Chinese medicine experts and Chinese medicine products cannot cope with the current need. There is a shrinkage of Chinese medicinal products; (iii) The training system of Chinese medicine experts fails to produce sufficient experts; and (iv) the traditional concepts and techniques fail to be properly developed (Lee, 2016).

Under the regulatory document being prepared, important issues include the following:

(i) Further support to include Chinese medicine as part of the Medical Insurance System.
(ii) Support non-government organisations and groups to provide Chinese Medicine Services in the form of hospitals, clinics and related structures, giving them encouragements comparable to modern medicine facilities.
(iii) Improve the qualification system for Chinese medicine experts so that proper qualifications could be accepted through unique scrutiny assessments outside institutional arrangements.
(iv) Improve the management details related to Chinese Medicine Services.
(v) Support innovative development of Chinese medicine productions.
(vi) Re-examine the related education system, give more emphasis on the traditional concepts and intensify the clinical training which could include apprenticeship.
(vii) Support the cultural aspect of Chinese medicine.

With the Legislation completed, it is expected that Chinese medicine in China would face a new era of innovative development.

References

Bivins, R. (2008). *Alternative Medicine? A History*. Oxford University Press, New York.

Cheng, Y.C. and Sze, D.M.Y. (2015). Globalization of Chinese medicine. In: *A comprehensive guide to Chinese medicine*. World Scientific Publisher, Singapore.

Jonas, W.B. (1998). Alternative medicine — learning from the past, examining the present, advancing to the future. *JAMA* **280**(18), 1616–1618.

Lee, S.K. (2016). Legislation for Traditional Chinese Medicine. *J. People's Congress of China* **1**(1), 33.

Leung, P.C. (2008). Debate on Chinese medicine. *J. Chin Med Ethics* **21**(6), 22–25.

Leung, P.C. and Wong, M.W. N. (2002). A critical analysis of professional and academic publications on Traditional Chinese medicine in China. *Am. J. Chin. Med.* **30**, 177–181.

Ministry of Health, People's Republic of China (MOH, China) (1995). *Traditional Chinese Medicine Services.* Ministry of Health, Peoples' Republic of China.

National Centre for complementary and Integrative Health (NCCIH) (2009). *Traditional Chinese Medicine: In Depth. March 2009,* Publication ID: D428. Available at: https://nccih.nih.gov/health/whatiscam/chinesemed.htm.

Singapore Ministry of Health (MOH, Singapore) (1995). *Traditional Chinese Medicine: A Report by the Committee of Traditional Chinese Medicine.* Ministry of Health, Singapore.

Stone, R. (2008). Lifting the veil on Traditional Chinese medicine. *Science* **319**(5864), 709–710.

Wong, T.W., Wong, S.L. and Donnan, S.P. (1993). Traditional Chinese medicine and Western medicine in Hong Kong: A comparison of the consultation processes and side effects. *J. Hong. Kong. Med. Assoc.* **45**, 278–284.

Xu, Q.Y. (2001). Medical education in China. In: *Proceedings on Health Care, East and West, Moving Into the 21st Century,* Harvard.

Chapter 10

Medicinal Herbs Used in Ayurveda and Chinese Medicine

Ping-Chung Leung and Edmond Au Wai-Chun

Abstract

The Ayurveda and Chinese Medicine share one common practice of prescription, *viz.* using multiple herbs in combination. Chinese medicine owns the classical guideline for the formulation of herbs, the Ayurveda system uses multiple herbs to counteract different aspects of observable symptoms, guided by rather rigid concepts.

This chapter would select a number of commonly used medicinal herbs in Ayurveda, and then look up their equivalents in the Chinese Pharmacopeia to illustrate the similarities and differences.

Keywords: Ayurveda; Chinese Medicine; Herbal Formulations.

10.1 Introduction

All the systems of traditional medicine (TM) rely heavily on medicinal herbs for the treatment of varieties of conditions. The Ayurveda and Chinese medicine share one common practice of prescription, *viz.* using multiple herbs in combination. Herbal formulations are favoured instead of single herb applications. Chinese medicine owns the classical guideline for the formulation of herbs since over 2,000 years ago: so that one herb in the formula in identified as the leading component (the Emperor), to be supported by the next important herb (the General) and other facilitators (the Ambassador and Warriors). If one single herb only is used, it must be known for and be useful for multiple functional purposes. On the other hand, the Ayurveda system uses multiple herbs to counteract different aspects of observable symptoms, guided by rather rigid concepts. Hence, similarities between the two systems in the use of medicinal materials do exist with regard to broad principles. Nevertheless, the traditional influences are so different that the same herb is often found to be used for widely diverged clinical purposes.

This chapter would select a number of commonly used medicinal herbs in Ayurveda, and then look up their equivalents in the Chinese Pharmacopeia to illustrate the similarities and differences.

10.2 *Hui Hui Yao Fang*

The *Hui Hui Yao Fang* is probably the oldest classical Arabic script that gives a properly documented account of medicinal herbs used in China before and after the Han Dynasty. The incomplete text of *Hui Hui Yao Fang* with missing chapters contains description of herbs and herbal formula shared during those ancient days between China and the Islam Sovereignties and India. This book which is equivalent to a pharmacopeia today could give a reliable idea about the herbs being used in the two systems (Kong and Chen, 1996).

Hui Hui Yao Fang is a formulary of 36 chapters with unknown authors. It was published at the end of the Yuen Dynasty in the 14th century. Unfortunately, only four chapters are available in full texts for academic study.

Analysis of the contents gives some basic idea about the nature of the medicinal herbs and their utilisations during those early days. Counting the number of times that herbs of different origins have been cited in the ancient formulary, it is found that Chinese herbs citations appeared about 2,500 times, Arabic herbs 1,800 times and foreign herbs 500 times. There is no distinction made between Arabic, Indian or foreign categories. Expectedly, many of those in the non-Chinese category could be of India origin. What this historical formulary offers us is that herbal medicine used in Traditional Chinese Medicine (TCM) contains a substantial among of material imported from outside China along the "silk-route" which includes India from Southwest, and Persian from the West.

About a century later, the most important Chinese classic on medicinal plants, "Compendium of Materia Medica" (*Ben Cao Gang Mu*) was compiled in the Ming Dynasty. Many of the plants listed are in fact imported from India and an overall one quarter are considered to be introduced from outside to China.

10.3 Comparing Ayurveda and Chinese Medicinal Plants

A number of commonly used Ayurveda herbs are chosen to compare and contrast with the same herbs used in (TCM).

No.		Ayurveda	Chinese medicine
1	*Abroma augusta (L)*		昂天蓮
	Family name:	Sterculiaceae	
	Common name:	Devil's cotton	Devil's cotton, Watery flax
	Sanskrit/Chinese:	*Pishach Karpas*	*Ang Tian Lian*
	Habitant:	Heights of 3,000–4,000 ft., wild as well as planted	Forrest land and slopes, south & south-west China
	Chemical composition:	resinous substances, carbohydrates, alkaloids, magnesium in hydroxy-acids	Maslinic acid; α-amyrin, vanillic acid; caffeic acid
	Properties:	Pungent, strong, kashaya	Pungent, bitter
	Medical uses:	Menstrual disorders/Gonorrhea	Soft tissue inflammation also topical use
2	*Aconitum heterophyllum Wall*		草烏頭
	Family name:	Ranunculaccae	
	Common name:	Indian Atis	Chicken poison; poison father; heart-breaking grass & many others
	Sanskrit/Chinese:	*Ativisha, Vishra*	*Cao-Wu Tou*
	Habitant:	Northwest India, altitude 15,000 ft.	Shrubs over slopes all over China
	Chemical composition:	Amorphous alkaloid atisine, aconitic acid, tannic acid	Aconitine; talatisamine; songorine, etc.
	Properties:	Bitter, digestive, cool	Pungent, bitter, hot poisonous
	Medical uses:	Mouth disorder/ Fever/bronchitis/ vomiting, gastritis/diarrhoea/ boils/acne	Analgesia; anaesthetic; cardio-toxic

(*Continued*)

(*Continued*)

No.		Ayurveda	Chinese medicine
3	*Achyranthes aspera L*		土牛膝
	Family name:	Amaranthaceae	
	Common name:	Prickly chaff flower	Native cow's knee
	Sanskrit/Chinese:	*Kinihi, Mayurak*	*Yun Niu Xi*
	Habitant:	Wild, grows all over India prosper in wet season	In wilderness and foot paths in South China
	Chemical composition:	High level of potassium	Ecdysterone; I-nokosterone
	Properties:	Anti-helminthic, blood purifier	Bitter; smooth
	Medical uses:	Migraine/tooth ache/eye disorder/ breathlessness/diarrhoea/ stomach disorder/ulcers/ infections	Diuresis; arthritis; swelling circulatory stagnation
4	*Aconitum ferox Wall*		烏頭屬
	Family name:	Ranunculaceae	
	Common name:	Monk's hood	Boat head
	Sanskrit/Chinese:	*Vatsanabha, Amrit*	*Chuan Kui Wutou*
	Habitant:	Himalayan region, heights 10,000–15,000 ft.	High altitude slopes near Himalayas
	Chemical composition:	Aconite, poisons	Aconites, poisons
	Properties:	Pacifies *tridoshas*, enhance potency	Pungent, hot, poisonous
	Medical uses:	Fever/diabetes/dysuria/pain/ swelling	Hepatitis, viral infections, analgesia, anaesthetic
5	*Acorus calamus L.*		水菖蒲
	Family name:	Araceae	
	Common name:	Sweet flag root	Muddy Tsung-Poo
	Sanskrit/Chinese:	*Vocha, Ugragandha*	*Tsung-Poo*
	Habitant:	From Europe, Asia, Himalayan region heights of 6,000 ft.	High grounds; Tibet
	Chemical composition:	Volatile oils painine, camphene, kalmanol, ekorine, starch, oxalates	Oils
	Properties:	Pungent, cool	Bitter, mild, dry
	Medical uses:	Headache/throat pain/epilepsy/ abdominal disorder/diabetes/ dysuria	Analgesic; gastro-tonic

(*Continued*)

(*Continued*)

No.		Ayurveda	Chinese medicine
6	*Aegle marmelos L. Correa*		木橘
	Family name:	Rutaceae	
	Common name:	Bael fruit	Wood tangerine
	Sanskrit/Chinese:	*Bilva, Sriphal*	*Mu-jud*
	Habitant:	Ancient Indian tree, holy	Highland tree
	Chemical composition:	Tannic acids, volatile oil, marmalosin	Volatile oils
	Properties:	Warm, cures *kapha*; *vata*; binds blood	No description
	Medical uses:	Headache/superficial infections/tuberculosis/abdominal pain/bowel syndromes/diabetes/dysuria/jaundice/weakness	Diarrhoea; eye tonic (topical)
7	*Aloe vera L. Burm*		蘆薈
	Family name:	Lilliaceae	
	Common name:	India aloe	Jelly grass
	Sanskrit/Chinese:	*Ghritkumarika, Sthool dala*	*Lu Hui*
	Habitant:	All over India	South China
	Chemical composition:	Glucosides, barbiloine, resin	Aloin, barbaloin
	Properties:	Pungent, cooling, bitter, cures *pitta*	Bitter, cold
	Medical uses:	Headache/eye disorders/bronchitis/abdominal pain/dysuria/diabetes/jaundice/arthritis/ulcers	Cough, haemoptysis
8	*Allium cepa L.*		洋葱
	Family name:	Liliaceae	
	Common name:	Onion	Jade grass
	Sanskrit/Chinese:	*Palandu, Yavneshth*	*Yan Con*
	Habitant:	All across India	Cultivated
	Chemical composition:	—	Citric acid
	Properties:	Vegetable, hot, pungent, unctuous, pacifies *vata*, enhance *pitta* and *kapha*	Vegetable, pungent
	Medical uses:	Cough/asthma/abdominal pain/improves sleep/diarrhoea	Health food, anti-infection

(*Continued*)

(*Continued*)

No.		Ayurveda	Chinese medicine
9	*Alangium salvifolium L. Wang*		土壇樹
	Family name:	Alangiaceae	
	Common name:	Alu Retis	Chinese *Azalea*
	Sanskrit/Chinese:	*Ankol, ankot*	*Bai Jiao gen*
	Habitant:	Scrub in forests, dry land high altitude	Scrub on slopes
	Chemical composition:		Venoterpine, anbasine
	Properties:	Improves *pitta*, purgative	Pungent, bitter, poisonous
	Medical uses:	Diarrhoea/Asthma/vomiting/fever/ poison	Joint pain, rheumatism
10	*Amomum subulatum Roxb*		香豆蔻
	Family name:	Zingiberaceae	
	Common name:	Greater Cardamom	*Jiu Kor-la*
	Sanskrit/Chinese:	*Brihadela, Sthulaila*	*Xian Dou Kou*
	Habitant:	Cooking material, wild in Himalayan regions	Woodland of 1,000 m altitude
	Chemical composition:	Fragrant oil contains cinial	Subulin; cardamonin, γ-terpinene
	Properties:	Suppresses *vata, Kapha*, enhances pita antipyretic	Pungent; warming
	Medical uses:	Oral problems/asthma/digestion/ dysuria/fever/diarrhoea	Gastro-tonic; cough
11	*Calotropis procera R.*		白花牛角瓜
	Family name:	Asclepiadaceae	
	Common name:	Swallow wort	Asthma tree
	Sanskrit/Chinese:	*Ark, Kshiraparna*	*Niu-jiu Kua*
	Habitant:	Dry barrier high ground	Hilly high ground, South China
	Chemical composition:	Poison, mandaralban	Calotropin, uscharitin, amyrin
	Properties:	Purgative, gastro-tonic	Bitter, poisonous
	Medical uses:	Infections/*pain/epilepsy/cough/ jaundice/arthritis/parasites*	Cough, asthma
12	*Adhatoda zeylanica Medik*		鴨嘴花
	Family name:	Acanthaceae	
	Common name:	Malabar nut	Fracture plant
	Sanskrit/Chinese:	*Vasak, Sinhasya*	*Ya Jui Hua*

(*Continued*)

(*Continued*)

No.		Ayurveda	Chinese medicine
	Habitant:	Heights of 1,200–4,000 ft., Stone rocky soil	Warm sandy grounds
	Chemical composition:	Alkaloids, vasa acid, resins, oils, carbohydrates	Magnolia terpines
	Properties:	Nourishes blood, cures *Kapha, pitta*	Bitter, pungent, warming
	Medical uses:	Headache/epilepsy/asthma/diarrhoea/eczema	Promote circulation, analgesia, bone injuries, arthritis
13	*Papaver somniferum L*		罌粟
	Family name:	Papaveraceae	
	Common name:	Poppy	*Ya-pien*
	Sanskrit/Chinese:	*Ahiphen*	*Yin-su*
	Habitant:	Cultivated	Cultivated
	Chemical composition:	Carbonic acids, resin, carbohydrates	Protopine; sanguinarine, cryptopine
	Properties:	Addictive	Sweet; soothing; addicting
	Medical uses:	Pain/Diarrhoea	Pain, diarrhoea
14	*Apium graveolens L.*		旱芹
	Family name:	Apiaceae	
	Common name:	Celery	Celery
	Sanskrit/Chinese:	*Ajmoda, Karvi*	*Han Cai*
	Habitant:	Cultivated	Cultivated
	Chemical composition:	Apiloa oil, albumen	Rorifamide, rorifone
	Properties:	Suppress *Kapha, vata,* elevates *pitta*	Warming, pungent
	Medical uses:	Pain relief/Asthma	Cough, food
15	*Trachyspermum ammi Sprague*		阿育魏實
	Family name:	Apiaceae	
	Common name:	Ajowan	*Ajowan*
	Sanskrit/Chinese:	*Yawani, Ajmodika*	*A Yu wei Shi*
	Habitant:	Flowering scrub	North, West China grassland
	Chemical composition:	Volatile oil, thymol	Thymols

(*Continued*)

(*Continued*)

No.		Ayurveda	Chinese medicine
	Properties:	Promotes *pitta*, warm	Pungent, bitter, warming
	Medical uses:	Cold/ cough/disinfect/ worms/ dysuria/flu	Analgesia, gastro-tonic
16	*Hyoscyamus niger L.*		莨菪子
	Family Name:	Solanaceae	
	Common name:	Henbane	
	Sanskrit/Chinese:	*Paarseek, Yawani*	*Tian Xian Zi.* Toothache Seed
	Habitant:	Heights of 8,000–10,000 ft.	Lowland Scrub
	Chemical composition:	Hyoscyamine, hyoscine, atropine	Atropine, Scopolamine
	Properties:	Calming, relax mind	Analgesic, sedative
	Medical uses:	Pain/arthritis/hysteria	Pain, toothache, epilepsy
17	*Anacyclus pyrethrum DC*		除蟲菊
	Family name:	Asteraceae	
	Common name:	Pellitory root	*Chrysanthemum cinerariae*
	Sanskrit/Chinese:	*Aakaraabh*	White flower insecticide
	Habitant:	From Greece, rainy season	Cultivated
	Chemical composition:	Volatile oil, inulin	Cinerin I & II Pyrethrin
	Properties:	Energises, stores body fluid	Bitter, cold
	Medical uses:	Headache/hysteria/fever/cough	Insecticide; anti-parasite
18	*Achyranthes aspera L.*		土牛膝
	Family name:	Amaranthaceae	
	Common name:	Prickly chaff flower	*Yun Niu Xi*
	Sanskrit/Chinese:	*Kinihi, Mayurak*	Hook gross
	Habitant:	All over India	Wild land & road side
	Chemical composition:	High potassium	Ecdysterone. L nokosterone Oleanolic acid
	Properties:	Cures *vata*, derive plant	Bitter, mild
	Medical uses:	Pain/asthma/gastric ailments/ ulcer	Boils, ulcers, muscleache
19	*Clitorea ternatea L.*		蝶豆
	Family name:	Papilionaceae	
	Common name:	Butterfly pea	Wild sweat potato

(*Continued*)

(*Continued*)

No.		Ayurveda	Chinese medicine
	Sanskrit/Chinese:	*Asfota, Giri Karni*	Butterfly pea
	Habitant:	Creeper in gardens	Tropical cultivation
	Chemical composition:	Carbohydrate, oil	Sterols, coumarin
	Properties:	Cures *tridoshas*, cooling	Stabilising, sweat
	Medical uses:	Headache/asthma/infection	Cough; asthma; boils
20	*Terminalia arjuna (Roxb) Wight*		三果木
	Family name:	Combretaceae	
	Common name:	Arjuna	
	Sanskrit/Chinese:	*Arjuna, Sambar*	*San Guo Mu*
	Habitant:	80 ft. talk tree in forests	Forest tree
	Chemical composition:	Bark: calcium carbonate, sodium	Arjunic acid, terminic acid
	Properties:	Cures *kapha, Pitta*, promotes circulation	Sweet, stabilising
	Medical uses:	Infection/Heart problems/Urinary problems: ulcers	Anti-inflammation
21	*Oroxylum indicum L.*		木蝴碟
	Family name:	Bignoniaceae	
	Common name:	Sword fruit	Rotten cloth
	Sanskrit/Chinese:	*Shyonak*	*Mu Hu Die*
	Habitant:	15–25 ft. tree, use root	Forest tree
	Chemical composition:	Flavon, resin	Oroxin A, Baicalein Benzoic acid
	Properties:	Bitter, warm	Bitter, mildly cool
	Medical uses:	Dysentery/asthma/ malaria/ arthritis	Stomachache; bronchitis blurred vision
22	*Premna latifolia Roxb*		大葉豆腐柴
	Family name:	Verbenanceae	
	Common name:	Nil	Nil
	Sanskrit/Chinese:	*Takeerna*	Nil
	Habitant:	Northern India, hills of 5,000 ft.	Scrub
	Chemical composition:	—	Phenolic oil

(*Continued*)

(*Continued*)

No.		Ayurveda	Chinese medicine
	Properties:	Warm blood	Nil
	Medical uses:	Heart/dyspepsia/allergy	Cooking
23	*Ocimum sanctum L*		羅勒
	Family name:	Lamiaceae	
	Common name:	Holy basil	Holy ocimum
	Sanskrit/Chinese:	*Vrirda, Tulsi*	Nine Levels Pagoda
	Habitant:	Grown medicinal plant	Cultivated
	Chemical composition:	Volatile oil	Carotene; sterol; ursolic acid
	Properties:	Polypotent, *Kapha vata*	Warm, bitter
	Medical uses:	Polypotent "holy plant"/ pneumonia/malaria/typhoid	Headache, asthma analgesic
24	*Phyllanthus Amarues*		葉下珠
	Family name:	Euphorbiaceae	
	Common name:	Indian gooseberry	Wild gooseberry
	Sanskrit/Chinese:	Bhoomyaamalakee	Wild gooseberry
	Habitant:	Hotter part of India	Tropical Scrub
	Chemical composition:	Lignans	Lignans
	Properties:	Cooling effects, cures *pitta*	Cool; stabilising
	Medical uses:	Jaundice/supports liver	Liver inflammation; gall stones
25	*Cannabis sativa L*		火麻
	Family name:	Cannabinaceae	
	Common name:	Indian hemp	*Da Ma*
	Sanskrit/Chinese:	*Bhanga vijaya*	Black hemp
	Habitant:	All over India	Scrub
	Chemical composition:	Resin, oil, sugar	Cannabinol
	Properties:	Enhances *Pitta*, bitter, warm	Poisonous, bitter
	Medical uses:	Diarrhoea/pain/asthma/ infections	Asthma; parasite disease stimulant; diarrhoea
26	*Foeniculum vulgare*		小茴香
	Family name:	Apiaceae Umbelliferae	
	Common name:	Fennel	*Fructus foeniculi*
	Sanskrit/Chinese:	*Mishreya*	茴香
	Habitant:	Cultivated	Cultivated

(*Continued*)

(*Continued*)

No.		Ayurveda	Chinese medicine
	Chemical composition:	Volatile oil, glycosides	Methyl chavicol, Volatile oils
	Properties:	Aroma, carminative	Sweet; bitter; warming
	Medical uses:	Anti-fungal/Anti-bacterial/ spasmolytic	Stomach fullness; analgesic; diarrhoea
27	*Terminalia chebula*		訶子
	Family name:	Combretaceae	
	Common name:	Chebulic	*Fructus chebulae*
	Sanskrit/Chinese:	*Abhaya, Pathya*	*Qing Guo*
	Habitant:	Hilly areas up to 5,000 ft.	Forest tree
	Chemical composition:	Tannin, amino acids, oil	Quinnin; galantosides
	Properties:	Dry, warm cures *pitta, tridoshas*	Bitter, Sour, Mild
	Medical uses:	Fever/cough/wounds/dyspepsia	Cough; diarrhoea; haemorrhoid
28	*Zingiber officinale*		生薑
	Family name:	Zingiberaceae	
	Common name:	Ginger	Ginger
	Sanskrit/Chinese:	*Adark*	*Jiang*
	Habitant:	Cultivated everywhere	Cultivated
	Chemical composition:	Carbohydrates, protein, oil	
	Properties:	Suppresses *kapha, vata*, warm	Warming; hot
	Medical uses:	Dyspepsia/pneumonia/dysuria/ pain	Vomit; cough; cold
29	*Glycyrrhiza glabra L*		甘草
	Family name:	Papilionaceae	
	Common name:	Liquorice	*Liquorice*
	Sanskrit/Chinese:	Madhuk	Sweet Grass
	Habitant:	Grown outside India	Cultivated
	Chemical composition:	Glycerryzin *Vata pitta shamak*	Glycerrhin, Liquiritin
	Properties:	Balance	Harmonising, poly potent
	Medical uses:	Multiple uses Eyes/voice/bronchitis	Multiple uses fits most formulations

(*Continued*)

(*Continued*)

No.		Ayurveda	Chinese medicine
30	*Piper longum*		蓽拔
	Family name:	Piperaceae	
	Common name:	Long pepper	Long pepper
	Sanskrit/Chinese:	*Pippali, Kana*	*Bi-Ba Geu*
	Habitant:	Import from Malaysia, Indonesia	From Persia now Cultivated
	Chemical composition:	Volatile oil, piperine, glycosides	Pepper salts
	Properties:	Suppresses *pitta, Kapha,* digestive	Warming; slight bitter
	Medical uses:	Heart problem/diarrhoea	Relaxant to smooth muscle

The Selection of the Ayurvedic and Chinese medicinal herbs for comparative interests has followed the following principles:-

(1) Commonly used herbs of general interest rather than those meant for specific utilisations.
(2) Ayurvedic herbs are mainly selected from three books: (i) Indian Herbs for Good Health (2), (ii) Indian herbal pharmacopoeia, and (3) Chinese Medicine and Ayurveda (4).
(3) Under the list of Indian Herbs for good health, 125 items are described. All the herbs have a large variety of health indication, varying from head to toe structurally and from daily ailments to severe pathologies. Careful scrutiny of the descriptions allow the choice of those with major and interesting properties to be selected.
(4) The selection of the 30 items has not considered their botanical or pharmacological natures. Neither is there special arrangement for particular medicinal uses.
(5) The more general clinical indications of the Ayurvedic category could resemble the Traditional Chinese uses. However, generally speaking, the Chinese prescriptions tend to be more concerned with specific clinical applications based on historical records (Dictionary of Chinese Medicinal Herbs, 2007; Chinese Herbal Medicine, 1998; Illustrative Collection of Chinese Herbs, 1990; Chinese Pharmacopeia, 2010).

10.4 Conclusion

Medicinal herbs have been contributing greatly in the health care of Indian as well as Chinese people. The clinical applications of the herbs have been based solely on the traditional records and beliefs. Similar clinical indications between Ayurveda and Chinese medicine appear logical and straightforward. Divergent situations might appear odd. Instead of making attempts to explain the discrepancies, researchers might pay special attention to the most popular herbs in common uses with common indications, to look for mechanisms of action and to hope for synergistic effects.

References

Chinese Herbal Medicine (中華本草) (1998). Shanghai Science and Technology Press, Shanghai.

Dictionary of Chinese Medicinal Herbs (2007). Science Publisher, Beijing.

Illustrative Collection of Chinese Herbs (1990). Peoples' Health Publisher.

Kong, Y.C. and Chen, D.S. (1996). Elucidation of Islamic drugs in Hui Hui Yao Fang: a linguistic and pharmaceutical approach. *J. Ethnopharmacol.* **54**(2–3), 85–102.

The Pharmacopoeia Committee of China (2010). *Chinese Pharmacopeia.* Chemical Industry Publish, Beijing.

Chapter 11

Ayurveda and Chinese Medicine Today: Joint Mission of the Two Asian Systems

Ping-Chung Leung and Debashis Panda

Abstract

Ayurveda and Chinese medicine are ancient, with over 3,000 years of age. Both have strong cultural and philosophical background. They have been providing practical services to the people of related regions ever since they are known and throughout their development. This chapter discusses the two Asian systems in their approach to health management and modern development.

Keywords: Ayurveda and Chinese Medicine; Holism; Harmony.

11.1 Introduction

The two Asian systems of health and medical treatment are put together and jointly discussed because of the obvious similarities. Both Systems are ancient, with over 3,000 years of age. Both have strong cultural and philosophical background: Ayurveda with Hinduism and Chinese Medicine with Buddhism and Taoism. They have been providing practical services to the people of related regions ever since they are known and throughout their development.

On the philosophical ideology, there are surprising similarities. They believe human and Nature are closely linked so that Nature affects the well-being of the individual and the physiological state of the individual must be analysed together with seasonal, environmental and weather influences.

Detection and diagnosis of what is going wrong depends on the detection of bodily changes through careful watching, listening and simple physical explorations. Anatomy and physiological functions are not known. Therefore, explanation of the result of detection of diagnosis would need a system of interpretation. Here comes the common spiritual part of both Ayurveda and Chinese medicine. The concept of life in both systems show strong spiritual links. The general vital state *prana* in Ayurveda and *Qi* in Chinese medicine of the individual is important. The vitality is affecting not only the prognosis but also the setting of the management plan. The vitality is the general reflection of the different interacting forces within the human body which need to be kept at a harmonious balance.

Both Ayurveda and Chinese medicine believe in Holism, i.e. taking the human bodily functions as a whole. Totally balanced bodily functions result in harmony and perfect health. The dysfunction of some parts leads to loss of the harmony manifested with different sets of disorders, syndromes and symptoms related to different organs. To remove the symptoms, not only are specific measures targeting towards the symptoms important, but it is also important to try to maintain the harmony of whole body. The simplest way of understanding the loss of harmony is to imagine that two opposing forces, one positive and one negative, are always acting against each other dynamically, so that under the perfect situation, positive and negative forces are at a balanced state. Otherwise, an excess or deficient state is the cause of symptoms and syndrome.

With regard to the management of diseases and ailments, both Ayurveda and Chinese medicine rely on medicinal herbs and manual therapy. Ayurveda, throughout the decades of changes, has maintained a much intense spiritual and religious practice of management while the Chinese counterpart is apparently adopting more and more deductive way of thinking.

Having so much similarities in their approach to health management, historically and culturally, Ayurveda and Chinese medicine should have a common mission in their modern development.

11.2 Challenges Imposing on Ayurveda and Chinese Medicine

The development and maturation of health care has followed the steps of science which is the result of the Industrial Revolution. Industrial Revolution happened in Europe, the rapid economic advances of which gradually led to colonialism. Countries and regions outside Europe, started to enjoy the benefits of science development only after their occupation by the European Nations. If biosciences and clinical science in the West have enjoyed just over 120 years of development, Asian Countries like India and China were allowed to follow the steps a few decades later. The impact of scientific advances including biosciences has been overwhelming. The facilitating stories about infection control and rescue of dying men have the most negative effects on traditional medicine (TM). Outcries for acquiring the modern scientific approach and giving up the traditional obsolete practices have been the logical outcome. In China, for instance, two major movements, one in the Qing Dynasty, another one in the early days of the Republic of China, to condemn Traditional Chinese Medicine (TCM) already occurred (Chang, 2006). Although the strong historical and cultural heritage would never have allowed elimination in the strict sense, TM would never be able to retain its originality.

The majestic power of science and technology have cast its overwhelming influence over all fields related to TM including education, service, research and commercial activities.

11.3 Education

In Education, traditional practitioners in Ayurveda and Chinese medicine could carry on taking their apprentices privately. However, to satisfy the demand on greater numbers of clinicians, standardisation and institutional teaching are logical needs. Such general mass programs need to observe the world trend. Traditional medical schools could not resist the addition of modern biosciences into the curriculum. It would also be the demand from the Public, the Health Authority and the students themselves, to include basic biosciences — Anatomy, Physiology and Pathology etc — into the traditional teaching. As a result, the newly trained traditional practitioners will be "brain-washed" by the bioscience information and gradually lose their ability to follow exactly what has been practised by the ancient masters. The current graduates of TM are therefore a "mix-breed" using scientific deduction and technical tools for both diagnosis and treatment, only that they also prefer adding traditional ways, that they are familiar with, as complementary or supplementary treatment. As more and more new drugs and devices are coming to market, the pressure on the traditional practitioners will be increasing accordingly.

11.4 Service

Traditional practitioners are giving excellent services to all those seeking their help. But in reality the mainline of service everywhere in the world, has been monopolised by modern allopathic medicine. Everyone would go to the hospital for emergencies and life-threatening treatment. Traditional practitioners are very careful not to admit that they better stay away from emergencies but they have to agree. Now that allopathic medicine has reached highly specialised practices with the establishment of many, many specialties, people would look for the specialty that they need rather than seeking simple advice and treatment from a clinician. Although traditional practitioner could claim that they are masters of certain specialty, they would be embarrassed if enquired about the same level of sophistication in their specialisation compared with allopathic medicine. Traditional practitioners could label themselves as generalists, which is acceptable only to a few. Before the day that a proper expert position is assigned to TM, the embarrassing situation probably continues to exist. This might not be ideal for the traditional practice in the long run.

11.5 Research

Since the current concept and practice of clinical research is very much a direct outcome of scientific exploration in the recent decades, one does not expect that TM would emphasise on research in the modern sense. The valuable classics and manuals of TM are full of case reports which give useful information about syndrome presentations and details of management. These are considered research records with lowest level of evidence. To go along the pathway of modern research on traditional clinical practice, hurdles are obvious and they present with excessive difficulties. Firstly, uniformity is a unique requirement for scientific research. When a uniform group of patients is required, both Ayurveda and Chinese medicine have difficulties because they consider every individual unique in his/her constitution and pattern and would not do well with uniform management. In the assessment of clinical progress, again uniform method and tools would be unacceptable. The actual treatment choice is also problematic if uniformity is insisted on. Moreover, quality control (QC) of medicinal herbs has never been satisfactory. If manual therapy is used, the practitioner could not convincingly stick to his/her technical applications.

Hence, either a brand new methodology needs to be established, or drastic compromises be accepted by the traditional group if research of acceptable quality is the desire.

11.6 Traditional Medicine Industry

The drug industry has always been in the hands of large multinational pharmaceuticals, without their commitment and investment, no sophisticated new drug could be produced after up-stream research. TM products (TMPs) range from dried herbs, herbal powders, granulations and proprietary medicine, none of which reaches the level of specific pharmaceuticals.

Since research on TM is complicated and restricted, the drug industry would give low priority to the traditional uses and variety of herbs. The vast need for herbal products has been satisfied by a large number of small enterprises which rely on either traditional connections to maintain a reasonable control of quality, or on "advertised quality". This obviously unsatisfactory situation is often the cause of safety issues and adulteration. Efficacy claim is not built on evidence-based research but on old classical reports and traditional folklore beliefs.

11.7 The Opportunity

Modern medicine is very much a reductional science. Specific target problems manifested as pathologies are identified before appropriate solutions could be found. Hypotheses are made, and using objective past data and specially designed methodology of research, they are gradually proven. Even negative results would serve subsequent attempts on related endeavours. Modern medicine has followed the pathway of development of modern science which has been so successful that any other channel of pursue would need to stand harsh criticism and it would not be easy at all for the alternative methodology to get recognition (Campion, 1993).

Asian TM has been inductive. It does not relate to very specific target, but instead, carries multiple foci of concern. It does not aim at solving a particular problem but aims at improving the general well-being of the individual by maintaining an effective balance between the various physiological functions.

Modern medicine commands the exactness which is the basis of all brilliant scientific achievements of the past 50 years. The exactness, however, has been criticised for being over-specific and as a consequence the general need of the individual might be neglected. While Asian Chinese medicine suffers the incapability of solving specific problems based on human biology, it follows a holistic approach with which the individual is kept balanced. The balanced, harmonious state would allow the individual to mobilise its biological reserves to take care of its own problems (Howick *et al.*, 2010).

While no one would have any doubt about the remarkable achievements in modern medicine: from specific removal of problems to accurate substitution of deficiencies and the recent genomic discoveries will probably lead to a total eradication of some pathologies and diseases, one could still remain dissatisfied, sceptical about the tread of development. The reductionist approach relies on accurate targets. Specialisation and subspecialisation thence become mandatory. The result of specialisation is over-specialization, which leads the way towards highly expensive services and the tendency of losing holistic care: patients are treated as "spare parts of a machine". The dilemma existing between modern achievements and patient disappointment because of the neglect of holistic care is one of the important reasons behind the popular support for alternative care and "off the counter" supply of health supplements (Eisenberg *et al.*, 1993).

While acknowledging the merits of the two different streams of medical service being provided *viz.* the modern and traditional systems, the unbiased medical scientists would agree, that, if the two divergent systems could be harmonised, a holistic care to promote a good physiological balance to allow spontaneous adjustment and strengthening of bodily defence, could supplement effectively the aggressive yet imperfect uni-focal modern medicine, which aims at the removal of specific problems.

Since 20 years ago bio scientists start to become aware of the limitations of modern Medicine. We have been overwhelmed with the successes of single target management which, however, fails to achieve 100% success. In fact 10–20% failures are common. How do we explain this phenomenon? Systems biology has found out that biological processes and pathological changes in fact are so complicated that many, many factors are involved: from organic, cellular, molecular and protein levels (CNRS, 1999). The influence of genomic predisposition and dynamic environment changes of both internal and external natures are other important areas contributing towards the changes. When one single pathology is successfully removed, and the patient recovers, we are just being lucky because the simplistic manoeuvre has been helped by hidden mechanisms. On the other hand, when in spite of all scientific methods, the results of treatment remains unfavourable, it is because the hidden mechanisms are not helping but instead, are disturbing the target treatment itself.

Scientists have started thinking about the holistic approach. Holistic approach is understood by the conventional scientist as the formation of a management plan that comprehensively tackle all pathological processes together. However, most of the time, we do not understand fully yet all the pathological processes.

The holistic approach for Asian medicine refers to supporting the whole person, maintaining a physiological balance, and an internal harmony so that while pathological processes are actively going on, yet the unaffected areas survive well and are helping to the maintain an effective defence system. In modern terms of understanding, the physiological state of harmony may mean a balanced immunological state which is expected to resist infection, suppress inflammation and maintains normal cellular and molecular activities. Such speculations and assumptions find perfect analogies in TM which does not claim target management but could provide holistic care. Of the different streams of TM, Chinese medicine possesses the largest volumes of classics, the richest collection of principles and theories and an immense number of records of medicinal material.

Moreover, acupuncture represents one area that is uniquely originated in China and is not found in other TM from other cultures including Ayurveda.

11.8 Upgrading Asian Traditional Medicine to International Level

Chinese medicine and Ayurveda give pride to all Chinese and Indian people because of their obvious link to Indian and Chinese culture and philosophy. The pride expands as people outside Asia are looking up to unique practices like Yoga and acupuncture and more and more people are using self-prescribed herbal supplements.

Upgrading Asian TM to an International level would certainly need research. Research on Herbal medicine in the past century has been focused on many aspects: from pharmacognosy, to QC, biological tests in the laboratory, authentication and clinical efficacies. Of these approaches much resource have been spent on the identification of the active herbal fractions and subsequently working out the chemical molecule responsible for the efficacy, with the obvious intension of developing an effective drug. There are a few successful examples in and outside Asia. One remarkable successful example in China was the discovery of the derivatives of Artemisinin (Qinghao) which currently is being used as standard treatment for malaria (Valecha and Tripath, 1997). Working on bioactive chemical components, using biochemical tests to identify molecular mechanism of bioactivity, and even exploration of toxicities, all belong to modern scientific technology, not TM. Strictly speaking, these methodologies of research are not related to the practice of TM, but have been successively utilised to cultivate valuable knowledge and practice from TM to enrich modern medicine.

As a matter of fact, drug discovery often finds its source from botanical material. Vincristine and Taxol for example, are extracted from the flower periwinkle and the bark of Yew trees respectively. The two cytotoxic drugs have become widely used (CNRS, 1999).

One has to realise the tremendous resources and facilities required for drug discovery. One also has to be aware of many other unsuccessful examples. Why are there limited numbers of successes in spite of so many attempts? Procedures of chemical isolation and deduction of the exact chemical molecule responsible for a certain bioactivity demands the endless efforts of the most advanced chemical laboratory and its technical team, followed by most expensive clinical trials.

There is a compromise, aiming at proving the efficacy of the herbal materials either as a gross extract, or using bioactivity fractionation techniques to isolate the bioactive groups of chemical compounds (Wong *et al.*, 2001).

The Efficacy Driven Approach has been discussed in detail in Chapter 7, here we give a simple exploration on the requirements:

(i) *Finding a way to harmonise TM and modern medicine*

Upgrading Asian medicine should not lead to the sacrifice of the basic philosophy and principles of TM. The principles of clinical treatment and the methodology of herbal formulation should be fully respected and applied. In the modern adoption of such principles, however, the technology of modern biomedicine could be utilised to improve the efficacy of treatment. Thus, the wise, selective choice of treatment method and herbal formulae, could be modified according to the current knowledge of pathology and diagnostics. Moreover the assessment of clinical results could follow the current requirements of good clinical practice, while background information would be generated from chemistry and biological platforms in the laboratories. Thus, Asian medicine enjoys a modernisation without losing its soul.

(ii) *Understand the details of clinical influences*

Efficacy is taken as a macroscopic, crude demonstration of the effects of the modality of treatment used for a clinical problem. Once preliminary evidences are established, more details of the clinical influences could be worked out. Further clinical studies included explorations on the objective events happening behind the improvement and the quality of life (Zhan and Lin, 2002).

(iii) *Understand the biological mode of action of the herbal formula*

This mainly involves laboratory tests of *in vitro* and *in vivo* nature. In the current era of molecular study, different animal models are usually needed and the biological pathways of action leading to the effects need to be defined.

(iv) *Understand the quality of the herbs*
All herbal formulae, once applied to solve a clinical problem would need to be further authenticated. One wants to get the best provision of the herb so that clinical effects could be guaranteed. Basic records of QC are established through chromatography studies (HPLC) which give the chemical profile, while the species details related to the origin of production are established with DNA finger printing during the filing of a voucher specimen.

Since consistent quality supplies of herbs are not available, every item should be subjected to screening and counter-checks, using standard extracts provided by the relevant academic institutions in China and India (Zhan and Lin, 2002).

(v) *Prepare for the improvement and optimisation of the formula*
Herbal formulae aim at additive and synergistic effects by mixing many herbs together. However, if the number of herbs is large, further development by manipulating the formula becomes difficult. Four to five herbs might be the maximal number in an innovative formula. When too many items are found in the classic formula, one could use modern concepts of pathology as guidelines of reduction. Since modern medicine works on direct targets, herbs advocated for direct actions could be eliminated because they could be substituted with modern medicine which should offer better direct actions. Those herbs that are understood to be immuno-modulating and promoting physiological balance, and be promotive on *prana* and *Qi*, on the other hands should be kept. In other words, when the major action of a herb is already covered by modern medicine, the herb could be eliminated. In the innovative creation of a formula or in the modification of a formula, the principles which Asian traditional practitioners had used for centuries — One major herb for main effect, others for enforcement and balance — could be respected.

(vi) *Rule out the possible interference with other pharmaceutical drugs being used*

When the mainline of clinical management is still modern medicine, the Asian medicine preparation is playing a supplementary role. It is important that the medicines being used should be tested against the pharmaceuticals being used, so that one could be certain that no adverse interactions are taking place. Before full scale popularisation takes place, the effective herbal preparation should be tested with the commonly used medications so as to prevent unfavourable interactions in other complicated platforms of Drug-herb interaction.

11.9 Conclusion

Ayurveda and Chinese medicine would stay as national prides. On the service side, it is already clear that they have a lot to offer in aging and chronic problems, pain control, neurological deficits and other situations when modern treatment does not satisfy all the needs. Whether Asian medicine would make greater international contributions in the field of medicine depends on whether proper research platforms could be built up to evaluate whether popular effective herbal preparations could be proven efficacious, and whether other measure could be proven excellent options of self-care.

While there should be no exclusion on the possibility of new drug discovery following the pharmaceutical's approach, more attention could be given on the health promotion side of food (herbs) supplements. The rich collection of herbs described in Asian classics that are used both as food and medicine, could be put under evidence-based clinical tests to show their supportive and preventive effects. With the proper investment and intellectual support, it seems likely that the key to the enrichment of allopathic biomedicine, which has not emphasised on the health maintenance and preventive manoeuvres from the individual, could be held in the hands of the enthusiasts on Asian medicine.

References

Campion, E.W. (1993). Why unconventional medicine?. *N. Engl. J. Med.* **328**, 282–283.

Chang, K.Y. (2006). Good-bye to Traditional Chinese Medicine. *Medicine and Philosophy.* **27** (4), 14–17.

Eisenberg, D.M. *et al.* (1993). Unconventional medicine in the United States — Prevalence, costs, and patterns of use. *N. Engl. J. Med.* **328**, 246–252.

Howick, J., Glasziou, P. and Aronson, J.K. (2010). Evidence-based mechanistic reasoning. *J. R. Soc. Med.* **103**, 433–441.

National Centre for Scientific Research France (CNRS). (1999). *Report on the Successes of Development of Drugs from Botanical Plants.* Special Report CNRS, France.

Valecha, N. and Tripath, K.D. (1997). Artemisinin: Current status in Malaria. *Indian J. Pharmacol.* **29**, 71–75.

Wong, W.N., Leung, P.C. and Wong, W.C. (2001). Limb Salvage in Extensive Diabetic Foot ulceration — A Preliminary Clinical Study Using Simple Debridement and Herbal Drinks. *Hong Kong Med. J.* **7**, 403–407.

Zhan, N.P. and Lin, R.C. (2002). The establishment of SOP for different Chinese Materia Medica in China [In Chinese]. *Res. Inform. Traditional Chinese Med.* **3**, 15–17.

Index

P

Q

R

S

T

www.ingramcontent.com/pod-product-compliance
Ingram Content Group UK Ltd.
Pitfield, Milton Keynes, MK11 3LW, UK
UKHW022103170926
8624IPUK00024B/53

9 789813 200333